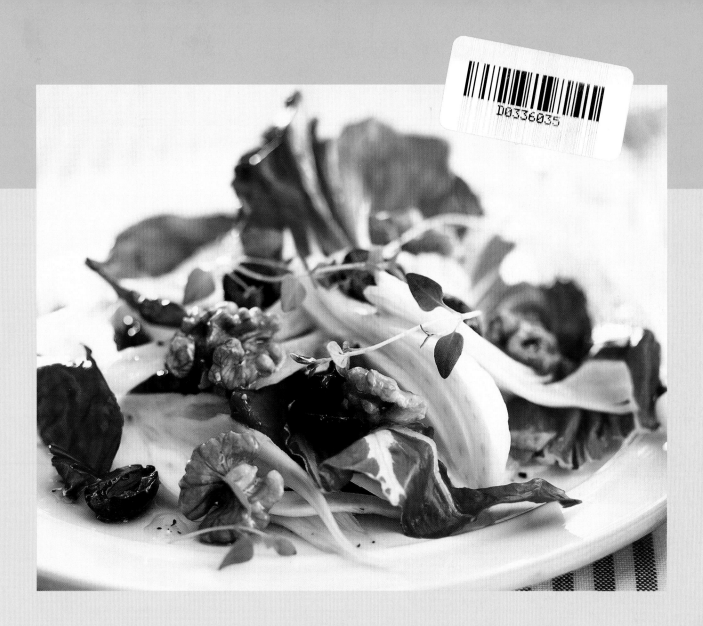

GREAT HEALTHY FOOD™
FOR THE
MENOPAUSE

ELAINE MYERS

CARROLL & BROWN PUBLISHERS LIMITED

First published in 2003 in the United
Kingdom by:

Carroll & Brown Publishers Limited
20 Lonsdale Road
Queen's Park
London NW6 6RD

Editor Caroline Smith
Art Editor Jacqueline Duncan
Photography Karen Thomas, Jules Selmes
Food Stylists Valerie Berry, Lorna Brash
Consultant Gaynor Bussell

Copyright © 2003
Carroll & Brown Limited

A CIP catalogue record for this book is
available from the British Library.
ISBN 1-903258-56-1

Reproduced by Colourscan, Singapore
Printed and bound in Italy by Eurolitho
First edition

The moral right of Elaine Myers to be
identified as the author of this work has
been asserted in accordance with the
Copyright, Designs and Patents Act
of 1988.

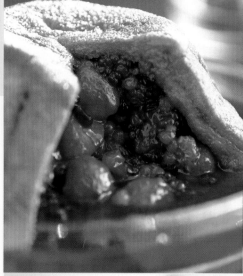
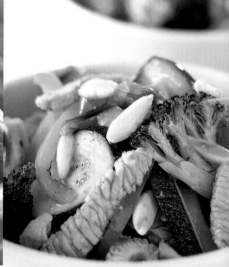
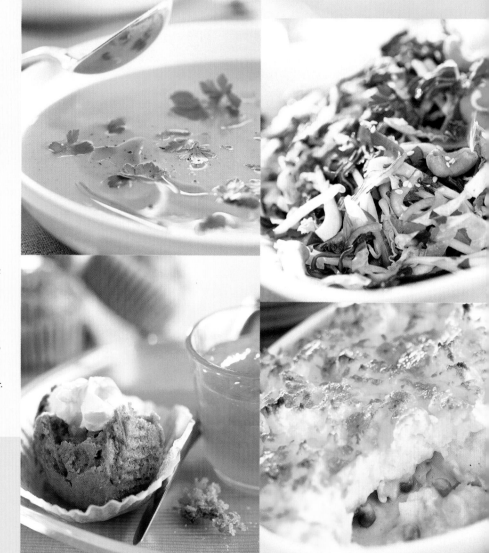

Contents

Introduction

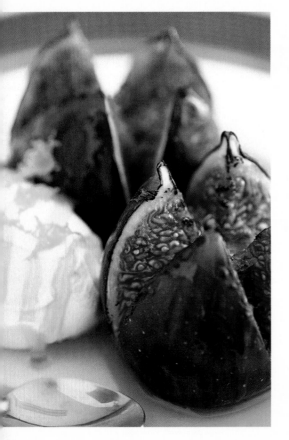

Women going through the menopause today are, in many ways, far more fortunate than their grandmothers, or even mothers. With more information about the menopause available and with their greater willingness to share experiences, women now have a better chance of relieving many menopausal symptoms. Probably one of the easiest ways for women to take control is to eat a healthy diet tailored to overcome or reduce menopausal symptoms. Eating the right foods also can help many other health issues that develop at this time of life, such as joint problems, thinning bones, weight gain and increased blood pressure. Even if you are receiving treatment from your GP for menopausal problems, a healthy diet can help the treatment work better. It may even enable you to reduce the medication you need, whether it's blood pressure tablets, osteoporosis drugs or hormone replacement therapy (HRT).

Nowadays, we are bombarded with information about food and nutrition, but some of it can be inaccurate. This book gives you information that is sensible, unbiased and accurate as well as delicious recipes that use the beneficial qualities of food. And since there is now an enormous variety of foods to choose from, all easily accessible at major supermarkets, it is easier than ever to modify our diets to address particular health issues. So there is really no excuse not to try out some of these recipes and do yourself a power of good! Although this is a cookery book designed for women going through the menopause, it doesn't mean that people of all ages can't eat the dishes. This book aims to give ideas for nutritious meals that are suitable for the whole family – whatever their sex or age. And research has shown that phytoestrogens (plant oestrogens) derived from food may be of benefit to younger women as well as to men of all ages.

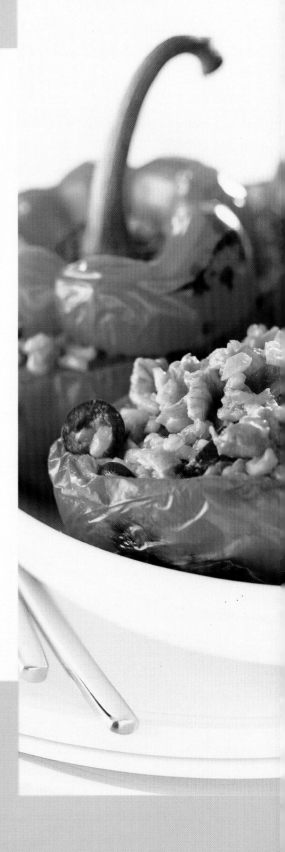

If you love food, are experiencing the menopause and want a healthy body, then this is the book for you. The recipes included can help reduce a wide range of symptoms because many of the ingredients used contain nutrients and other elements, such as phytoestrogens, known to help menopausal problems. You don't have to eat tofu burgers forever, you can still enjoy delicious food.

NATURAL HRT
Phytoestrogens are naturally occurring hormones, found in plant foods, that mimic the female hormone, oestrogen. However, they do this only when women's own oestrogen levels fall in menopause. They can help with several symptoms, especially hot flushes, and may also reduce the risk of osteoporosis, as well as several cancers and heart disease. Unlike HRT, phytoestrogens are believed not to increase the risk of breast or endometrial cancer.

Currently, there is much research being done on phytoestrogens with very positive results. New research shows that they may also help with cognitive function after the menopause. Phytoestrogens that come from food seem to work better than those taken in the form of a supplement. They also seem to work more efficiently if your diet is high in fish oils and seeds that contain the Omega 3 fatty acids. Phytoestrogens are found in many fruits, vegetables, seeds and beans, but occur in the highest concentrations in soya products, including tofu and soya milk, and in chick peas, linseeds and wheat bran.

PROTECTING YOUR BONES
During the menopause, women's bones lose calcium at an accelerated rate, so anything that helps to alleviate this is important. Women need to keep up some

WHAT IS THE MENOPAUSE?
Also known as the climacteric, this occurs when the ovaries cease to produce the hormone oestrogen. The winding-down phase is known as the peri-menopause, and it can go on for a few years and may be accompanied by irregular periods and the start of recognised menopausal symptoms. The true menopause occurs when periods stop completely because of the lack of oestrogen. It occurs at an average age of 51 years, but may happen between the ages of 45 and 55. Younger women can be affected too, if they have a naturally premature menopause or if a premature menopause is brought on by surgery, when both ovaries are removed.

The most common symptoms of declining oestrogen levels are osteoporosis, hot flushes, night sweats, anxiety, depression, panic attacks, declining libido, vaginal dryness, palpitations, bladder problems, ageing skin, lack of energy, joint pains, general aches and pains, weight gain, irritable bowel syndrome (IBS), headaches and changes in hair quality.

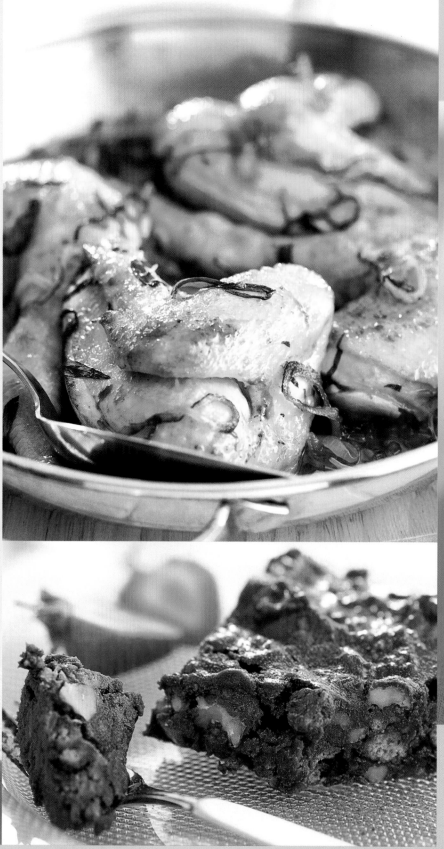

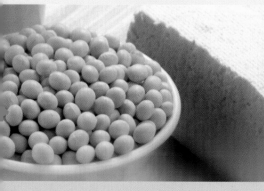

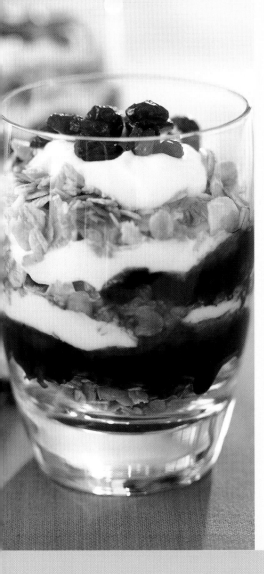

weight-bearing exercise, but diet can also play a big part. Calcium contributes about 1 kg to the average woman's body weight. As well as being vital in bone strength, it aids blood clotting, helps the nerves transmit signals, prevents muscle cramps and skin problems, and can help with insomnia, depression and cognitive impairment.

To provide the body with essential calcium, women need to eat calcium-rich foods, which include, milk, cheese, yogurt, fortified soya milk, tofu, sardines, dried fruit, beans and some seeds. In order to absorb calcium, women also need vitamin D, a fat-soluble vitamin found in oily fish, eggs and butter or margarine. Eating plenty of fruit and vegetables has also been shown to protect the bones, and phytoestrogens may be protective too. Too much salt and alcohol, however, are detrimental to bone health.

A Healthy Heart

Women's chances of suffering heart disease increase during the menopause. However, there are several ways you can decrease the risk. You could up your intake of phytoestrogens as these have been shown to have cardio-protective effects. You should use the healthier fats for cooking; olive oil or any oils and fats based on rapeseed oil have been found to be the most heart-protective. Rapeseed oil is best as it contains a high level of monosaturated fats and is rich in heart-protecting Omega 3 fats. Olive oil is also rich in monosaturated fats. Other seed and nut oils, such as walnut, sesame seed and flax (linseed) oil, are healthy because they tend to be monosaturated and/or rich in Omega 3. Use them for dressings as they retain their best nutritional benefits if not heated.

Sunflower oil, rich in polyunsaturated fats, is not too bad and may help lower harmful fats in the blood. However, too much polyunsaturated fat may cause oxidative damage to the body. You should avoid a diet high in saturated fats, such as lard, butter, cream and dripping, and cut out trans fats – the artificially hardened fats and oils often found in cheap pastries, pies and biscuits.

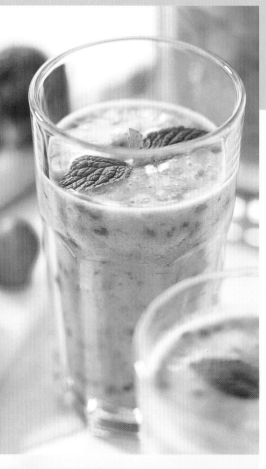

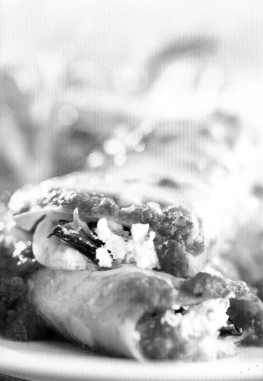

You also need to cut down your salt intake. Salt increases blood pressure, which in turn increases the risk of stroke and heart disease. The recipes in this book use the least salt necessary for flavour.

WATCHING YOUR WEIGHT

As you get older it tends to be harder to lose weight and oh so much easier to pile it on! Excess weight after the menopause can contribute to increased cholesterol levels and other harmful blood fats, raised blood pressure, an increased risk of several cancers, worsening joint problems and diabetes. Eating a well-balanced diet will help.

Fat intake is an important issue. Some oils are better for us than others (see p. 7), however all fats and oils, unless labelled as reduced fat, have the same number of calories – roughly 900 calories per 100 g or 45 calories per teaspoon! As fats are so calorie dense you need to keep your total fat intake down when watching your weight. Just make sure the fats and oils you do choose are the healthier variety.

However, you should not aim to be too thin. Women continue to produce some oestrogen after the menopause, but it is manufactured in the adipose (fat) tissue rather than in the ovaries. If you are too thin after the menopause, you will miss out on producing some of your own natural oestrogen, which may help to offset some menopausal symptoms. You'll also be at greater risk of suffering with osteoporosis.

THE BEST ADVICE ...

To sum it all up, the best advice, if you are going through the menopause, is to eat a wide variety of foods. This will ensure your body gets a mixture of all the nutrients it needs. To make the most of your food's flavour and get the maximum nutritional benefit, you should try and eat dishes that you have made yourself from really fresh ingredients – processed foods and 'ready meals' tend to use inferior ingredients and too much salt.

Eat lots of fruit and vegetables and use ingredients based on wholegrains and foods that have not had their fibre-rich outer layers removed. This ensures you get the maximum nutritional value from the food and fibre too – and helps you to avoid constipation and IBS. Eat a starch food with every meal, such as brown rice, pasta, wholegrain bread or cereal. This will regulate blood sugar effectively and ensure that you don't get too hungry before the next meal. Each main meal should also contain some protein and lots of vegetables or salad. A diet containing plenty of phytoestrogens may help to combat many menopausal symptoms.

NOTES TO THE COOK

In these recipes, the salt content has been kept to a minimum. If you must season with salt, try to use as little as possible. All cow's milk used is semi-skimmed, unless otherwise stated.

MENOPAUSAL SYMPTOMS	WHAT TO EAT AND WHAT TO AVOID
Hot flushes	Eat soya-based foods and linseeds. Use the herb, sage. Avoid too much spicy food, caffeine and alcohol.
Mood swings, anxiety & irritability	Eat foods high in magnesium such as brown rice, whole wheat, whole rye, beans, lentils and peas and green vegetables. Eat regularly and try to include a starchy food with each meal. Avoid too much caffeine, sugary foods and alcohol.
Insomnia	Avoid caffeine too late at night. Avoid eating a big meal late in the evening. Try a bedtime snack which contains some milk or yogurt and something starchy – such as natural yogurt and a banana, or crispbread with cottage cheese, or some hot milk and a low-fat biscuit.
Heavy bleeding	Eat an iron-rich diet to replace lost iron, such as red meat, green vegetables, beans and sardines.
Vaginal dryness	Eat soya products, such as tofu or soya milk, or linseeds, as they can replace lost oestrogen.
Osteoporosis	Eat calcium-rich foods, such as milk, cheese, yogurt, fortified soya milk, tofu, sardines, dried fruit, beans and some seeds. Eat foods rich in vitamin D, such as oily fish, eggs and butter or margarine. Foods rich in phytoestrogens may also help, such as soya products, chickpeas, linseeds and wheat bran.
Night sweats	Try sage taken as a tea at bedtime (3–5 leaves in hot, not boiling, water). Include sage leaves in cooking. Eat phytoestrogen-rich foods (see osteoporosis, above).
Ageing skin	Eat an anti-oxidant-rich diet containing plenty of fresh fruits and vegetables, wholegrains and seeds. Eat foods high in vitamin E, such as nuts, avocados, seeds and oily fish. Include essential fatty acids such as those found in vegetable oil, nuts and fish oils.
Depression	Eat a diet containing plenty of oily fish. If you drink a lot of alcohol, make sure your diet includes foods rich in B vitamins, such as meat, fish, eggs, milk and cheese and wholegrain cereals.
Joint pains	Eat oily fish and phytoestrogen-rich foods (see above).
Bloating	Reduce your salt intake – in your cooking, at the table and by avoiding too many processed foods. Drink plenty of fluid, especially plain water, to keep the kidneys working efficiently.
Constipation & IBS	Eat plenty of fibre derived from wholegrain cereals, fruit and vegetables. Drink at least 2 litres of fluid a day. Avoid too much caffeine and alcohol.

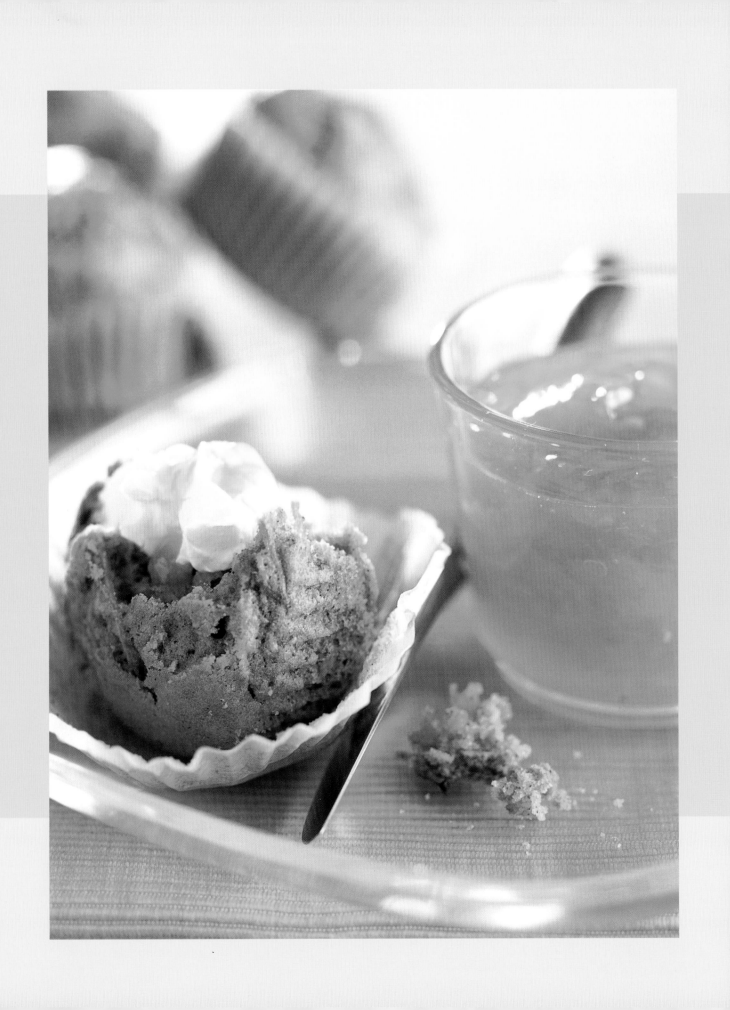

1

A Good Start

IT IS OFTEN SAID THAT
BREAKFAST IS THE MOST
IMPORTANT MEAL OF THE DAY.
HERE YOU'LL FIND PLENTY OF
DISHES – BOTH LIGHT AND
FILLING, SWEET AND SAVOURY
– THAT WILL SET YOU UP FOR
THE DAY AHEAD.

MANGO & PEACH SMOOTHIE

3 large ripe mangoes

5 ripe peaches

750 ml soya milk

750 ml orange juice

150 g plain live yogurt

Crushed ice, to serve

Serves 4

A great way to get your taste buds going in the morning, this is a smoothie with a totally tropical flavour, packed with vitamin C and other anti-oxidants. The live yogurt may help with gut health and boost immunity.

1   Peel the mangoes and peaches and remove the stones; discard. Chop the flesh roughly.

2   Place the fruit in a food processor or blender with the soya milk, orange juice and yogurt. Process until smooth then pour into glasses and add some crushed ice to serve.

PAPAYA & NECTARINE SMOOTHIE

You can use papaya and nectarines in this recipe. Just cut 2 ripe papayas in half and scoop out the seeds. Peel and chop the flesh. Prepare the nectarines in the same way as the peaches. Then put the fruit in a food processor with the liquids and yogurt – you could try using a blend of tropical fruit juices instead of orange juice.

COFFEE BANANA SMOOTHIE

4 teaspoons espresso coffee powder

100 ml boiling water

600 ml skimmed milk

250 ml soya milk

2 bananas

8 ice cubes

Ground cinnamon (optional)

Serves 4

This is ideal if you need an occasional caffeine treat. The banana contains potassium, which may help reduce blood pressure, and there are phytoestrogens in the soya milk.

1   Mix the espresso powder with the boiling water and then leave it to cool for 5 minutes.

2   Pour the skimmed milk and soya milk into a food processor or blender. Chop up the bananas and add to the milks. Pour in the cooled coffee and add the ice cubes.

3   Process for 30 seconds and then pour into 4 glasses. Serve immediately or chill for 20–30 minutes, until a little froth forms on the tops of the smoothies. Sprinkle with cinnamon to serve, if liked.

Very Berry Smoothie

Packed with berries – and phytoestrogens – this is a perfect drink for first thing in the morning. But you can also make it later in the day for that extra burst of fruity goodness.

1 Wash all the strawberries or berries. Hull any strawberries and trim any other berries. Drain and dry thoroughly and transfer to a food processor or blender. Peel the bananas and chop roughly; add to the food processor.

2 Add the yogurt, soya milk, linseeds and honey and process until smooth. Pour into glasses and chill for a few minutes, if liked, before serving, decorated with sprigs of mint.

750 g strawberries or a mixture of berry fruits

3 bananas

500 g plain live yogurt

750 ml soya milk

1 tablespoon linseeds

3 tablespoons honey

Sprigs of mint, to decorate

Serves 4

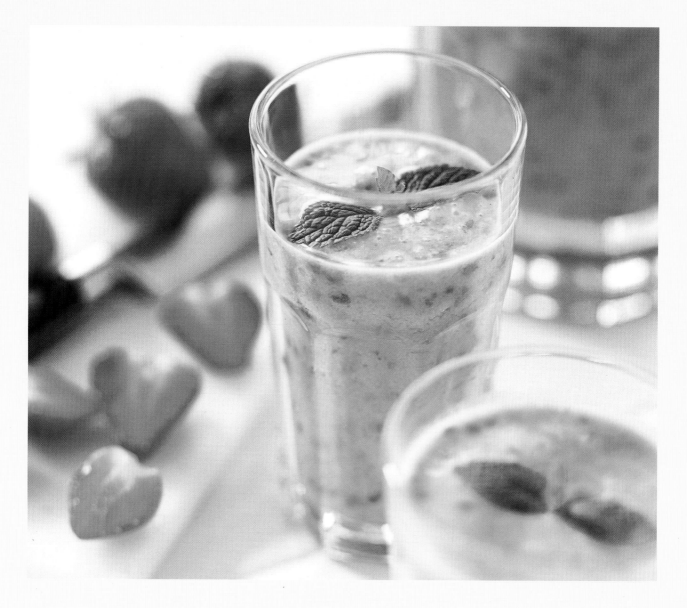

GRILLED PINK GRAPEFRUIT WITH NUTMEG & MAPLE SYRUP CRUST

2 large pink grapefruits

4 teaspoons maple syrup

4 tablespoons demerara sugar

½ teaspoon freshly grated nutmeg

Serves 4

A great way to start the day with a vitamin C boost, this is a delicious breakfast dish but would also make a good dinner-party starter.

1 Heat the grill to its highest setting. Peel the grapefruits and separate them into segments. Transfer the segments to a shallow flame-proof dish that's just large enough to hold them, packed into a single layer with no gaps.

2 Mix the maple syrup, sugar and nutmeg together and drizzle the mixture over the grapefruit segments. Place the dish under the grill and grill for 4–5 minutes until the sugar melts and begins to form a crust.

GRILLED CITRUS FRUITS WITH A ZESTY SYRUP CRUST
Why not try this dish with a mixture of different citrus fruits? To begin, mix 1 teaspoon grated orange zest, 1 teaspoon grated lime zest with 4 teaspoons golden syrup and 4 tablespoons soft light brown sugar. Then peel 1 clementine, 1 small orange and 1 ugli fruit and divide them into segments. Lay them out in a flameproof dish, as above, and cover with the zest, syrup and sugar mixture. Grill for about 5 minutes until the sugar melts. Don't allow the zest to burn.

BAKED BANANAS WITH NUTMEG & MAPLE SYRUP
The maple syrup and nutmeg combination works well with bananas. Preheat the oven to 200°C, gas mark 6. Lay out four separate squares of foil and place a peeled banana on each one. Drizzle 2 teaspoons of maple syrup over each banana then sprinkle each one with 2 teaspoons of demerara sugar. Grate a little fresh nutmeg over each banana then scrunch the foil loosely around each one and transfer to a baking tray. Bake for about 20 minutes until the bananas have softened.

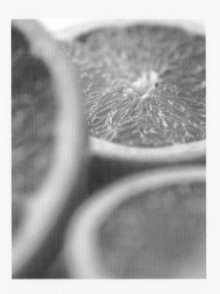

CARIBBEAN PORRIDGE

A new take on an old favourite, this makes a creamy, but low-fat breakfast. The oats help steady blood sugar and keep you satisfied until lunchtime. The soya milk provides some natural oestrogen.

1   Peel the papaya, cut it in half and scoop out the seeds; discard. Transfer the fruit to a food processor or blender and purée.

2   Mix the oats and desiccated coconut together in a saucepan. Stir in the soya and coconut milks and place the pan over medium heat. Bring the mixture to a boil, stirring all the time, then reduce the heat to low and continue to cook, stirring, for 5–10 minutes until the porridge reaches the consistency you prefer.

3   When the porridge is cooked, stir in the golden syrup and then transfer to individual bowls. Swirl the papaya purée into each serving.

1 large papaya

80 g porridge oats

50 g desiccated coconut

250 ml soya milk

375 ml coconut milk

3 tablespoons golden syrup

Serves 2–3

DRIED APRICOT PURÉE WITH CARIBBEAN PORRIDGE

This recipe works just as well with dried apricots. Place 150 g dried apricots in a saucepan with 200 ml orange or apple juice. Bring to a boil and then simmer for about half an hour until the dried fruit is soft. Allow to cool slightly before puréeing in a food processor or blender. Stir the purée into the cooked Caribbean porridge.

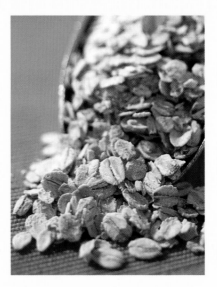

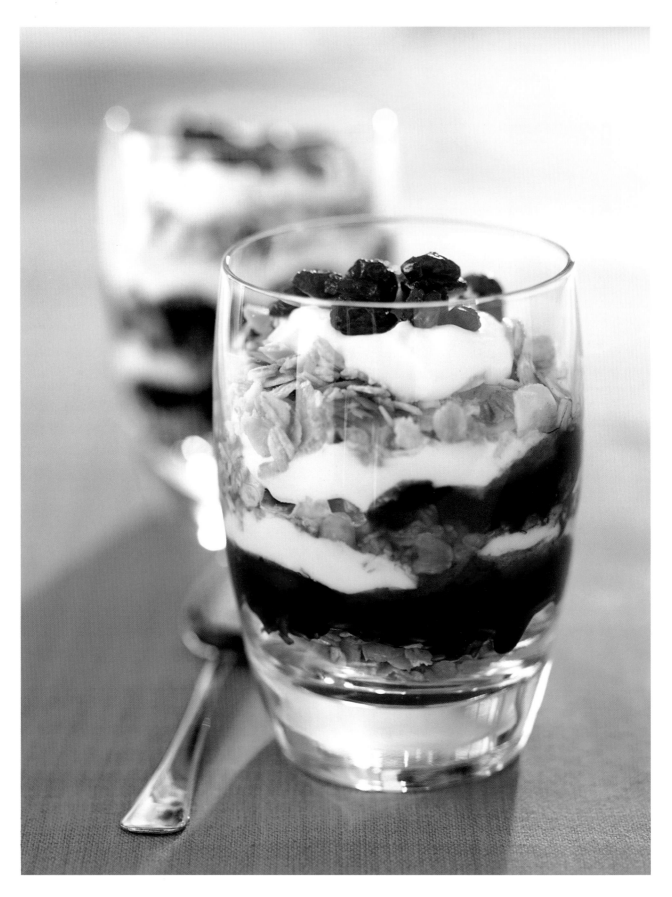

Vanilla Granola Breakfast Trifle

A delicious breakfast made up of layers of granola, fruit conserve and yogurt. It is very filling and provides long-lasting energy – great if you have a long gap between breakfast and lunch.

1 To make the granola, preheat the oven to 150°C, gas mark 2. Line a large baking tray with greaseproof paper. Mix the oats, almonds, sugar, salt and cinnamon together in a large bowl.

2 Stir the oil and honey together in a small saucepan and heat over medium-high heat, stirring, until quite hot. Remove from the heat and stir in the vanilla extract. Pour into the bowl with the oat mixture and stir well until all the dry ingredients are thoroughly coated.

3 Spread the mixture on the lined baking sheet and bake in the centre of the oven for 30 minutes. Leave to cool on the tray for 10 minutes and then pour into a bowl to cool completely – don't leave it any longer or it will stick to the greaseproof paper.

4 To assemble the dish, pour a couple of spoonfuls of cooled granola into the bottom of a tall glass. Add a tablespoon of the fruit conserve and then a couple of tablespoons of yogurt. Add another layer of the granola and then more fruit conserve and yogurt. Repeat to fill three more glasses. Top each one with a tablespoon of dried cranberries or cherries.

250 g oatmeal or porridge oats

60 g slivered or sliced almonds

30 g demerara or soft light brown sugar

¼ teaspoon salt

½ teaspoon ground cinnamon

50 ml rapeseed or sunflower oil

60 ml runny honey

2 teaspoons vanilla extract

500 g plain soya yogurt or plain Greek yogurt

8 tablepoons sugar-free blueberry or blackcurrant conserve

4 tablepoons dried cranberries or cherries

Serves 4

GRANOLA WITH MILK

The granola makes a delicious breakfast cereal in its own right, served with whatever kind of milk you prefer. If you like, mix a few tablespoons of raisins or sultanas in with the oat mixture after it has been baked. You can also make up a double amount of the granola and keep it for further breakfasts – it will keep for a week or two stored in an airtight container.

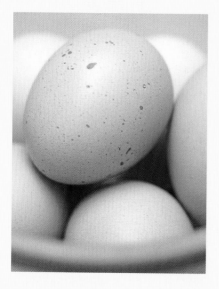

FRENCH-TOASTED BRIOCHE WITH FOREST BERRY SAUCE

A dish that makes use of the goodness of berries, which contain anti-oxidant flavonoids and vitamin C. Slices of brioche are dipped in egg, a source of protein, before cooking to give a crisp and tasty coating.

1 Thoroughly defrost the frozen berries, retaining any juices. Preheat the oven to 170°C, gas mark 3. Beat the eggs and milk together. Cut the brioche loaf into 5 cm-thick slices, discarding the heel.

2 Pour the egg mixture into a large shallow dish, big enough to take all the brioche slices in one layer. Place each slice in the mixture and turn it. Leave to soak for 5 minutes.

3 Meanwhile, transfer half of the berries with all the juices to a food processor or blender. Add the sugar; purée. Pour into a bowl and stir in the remaining berries.

4 Grease the base of a large non-stick frying pan with some butter. Place the pan over a medium-high heat and when it is hot, add enough brioche slices to fit in the pan and cook them for a couple of minutes on each side until golden brown. Continue until all the brioche slices are cooked, re-greasing the frying pan as necessary.

5 Transfer the brioche to a baking tray and bake in the middle of the oven for about 5 minutes until hot and crisp. Serve at once, topped with the berries.

250 g bag mixed frozen berries, such as blackberries, redcurrants and blackcurrants

3 eggs

100 ml milk

½ large brioche loaf

3 tablespoons caster sugar

Butter, for greasing

Serves 4

CARROT BREAKFAST MUFFINS

These light fluffy muffins are high in betacarotene and a great way to eat linseeds, with their oestrogenic properties. You can make these in advance but they are delicious warm. Serve with the optional cream cheese and jam, if liked.

1   Preheat the oven to 200°C, gas mark 6. Line 6 cups of a deep muffin tin with paper liners. Sift the flour, salt, bicarbonate, baking powder and cinnamon together into a large mixing bowl.

2   Break the egg into another mixing bowl and add the sugar and oil; whisk together. Stir the grated carrots, linseeds and orange zest into this mixture and then fold the sifted dry ingredients into it, a spoonful at a time.

3   Spoon the mixture into the prepared muffin cases and bake in the centre of the oven for 20–25 minutes, until golden. Leave to cool slightly in the cases.

4   To serve, break open the muffins while still warm and spread with a little cream cheese and jam, if liked.

125 g self-raising flour

½ teaspoon salt

¼ teaspoon bicarbonate of soda

¼ teaspoon baking powder

1½ teaspoon ground cinnamon

1 egg

55 g soft light brown or golden granulated sugar

100 ml rapeseed or sunflower oil

3 small carrots, finely grated

10 g linseeds

Grated zest of 1 orange

Low-fat cream cheese, to serve (optional)

Sugar-free apricot jam, to serve (optional)

Makes 6 muffins

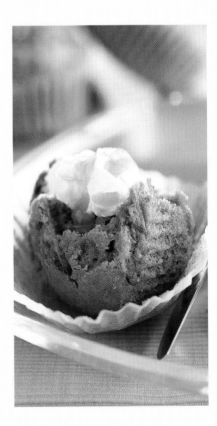

DAILY LOAF

25 g dark chocolate

100 g soya flour

100 g plain white flour

100 g porridge oats

100 g linseeds

50 g sunflower seeds

50 g sesame seeds

50 g flaked almonds

75 g dried cranberries

1 teaspoon ground mixed spice

100 g mixed dried fruit – such as sultanas, currants, raisins, apricots, cherries, peaches and figs

1 tablespoon black treacle

2 tablespoons cranberry, grape or apple juice

750 ml soya milk

Makes 18–22 slices

This light but moist loaf contains phytoestrogen-rich foods, such as linseeds, and so may go a long way to relieve many menopausal symptoms. A slice of this loaf will be broken down slowly by the body and so can also provide you with long-lasting energy.

1 Grate the chocolate into a large bowl. Add all the rest of the ingredients, except the fruit juice and soya milk, and mix well. Stir in the fruit juice and soya milk and leave to stand for 1 hour.

2 Preheat the oven to 190°C, gas mark 5. Line a 900 g loaf tin and a 450 g loaf tin with greaseproof paper. (Alternatively, use three 450 g loaf tins.) Spoon in the cake mixture until both tins are two thirds full.

3 Place the tins in the oven and bake the larger tin for 2 hours, the smaller one for 1½ hours. Test each loaf by inserting a skewer. When the skewer comes away completely clean, cook the loaves for another 10 minutes.

4 Leave the loaves to cool for 30 minutes in the tins before turning out on to a wire rack to cool completely. Cut into slices about 2 cm thick to serve.

STORAGE ADVICE

This loaf will only keep at its best for a few days, stored in an airtight container. It does, however, freeze well so it is worth making up several batches. Cut the loaf into slices and wrap individually before freezing. Since this loaf is packed with good things for the menopause, it also makes a perfect daily snack or treat as well as a filling breakfast bake. A few slices in the freezer will ensure you always have some of this delicious, healthy loaf to hand.

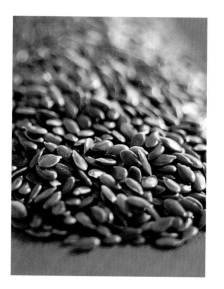

Banana & Cottage Cheese Topped Bagels

This makes a very filling breakfast dish, packed with energy. The sweetness of the bagels is perfectly teamed with the creamy topping and crunchy walnuts.

1   Place a cast-iron skillet or heavy-based frying pan over medium-high heat. When the pan is hot, add the walnuts and cook, stirring, for about 1 minute until the nuts give off an aroma. Set aside to cool.

2   Heat the grill to medium high. Split each bagel in half and place, cut side down, under the grill. Toast for a few minutes until golden then turn each one and toast for a few minutes more.

3   Put the tofu into a bowl and mash. Stir in the cottage cheese. Thinly slice the bananas and stir into the mixture with the cooled walnuts.

4   Place two bagel halves on each serving plate and top each one with the cottage cheese, tofu, banana and walnut mixture. Drizzle honey over each bagel half and serve.

50 g chopped walnuts

4 bagels

25 g soft silken tofu

150 g low-fat cottage cheese

2 large bananas

2–3 tablespoons runny honey

Serves 4

Smoked Salmon & Quark with Onion Bagels

Quark is a low-fat curd cheese that makes an excellent alternative to cream cheese. Team it with smoked salmon for a tasty savoury breakfast bagel.

1   Cut the smoked salmon into fine strips, about 3 cm long. Put the Quark in a bowl with the dill. Season with a little black pepper and beat together. Stir in the smoked salmon strips and chill for a few minutes to firm the mixture and let the flavours mingle.

2   Meanwhile, heat the grill to medium-high. Split each bagel in half and place, cut side down, under the grill. Toast for a few minutes then turn each one and toast for a few minutes more until golden.

3   Place two bagel halves on each serving plate and spread each one with the smoked salmon mixture. Sprinkle each one with snipped chives and serve with lemon wedges to squeeze over the top.

150 g smoked salmon

250 g tub Quark

1 tablespoon chopped fresh dill

Freshly ground black pepper, to taste

4 onion bagels

A few fresh chives, snipped, to serve

1 lemon, cut into quarters, to serve

Serves 4

Oven-baked Hash Brown with Tomato Gratin

1 large potato, cut into 2 cm cubes

1 sweet potato, cut into 2 cm cubes

300 g acorn squash, cut into 2 cm cubes

2 tablespoons olive oil

1 onion, finely chopped

2 cloves garlic, crushed

1 teaspoon caraway seeds

2 tablespoons paprika

2 beefsteak tomatoes

80 g fresh breadcrumbs

50 g Parmesan cheese, grated

3 tablespoons roughly chopped fresh parsley

Serves 4

A perfect weekend brunch dish, this hash brown is made of two different kinds of potato, mixed with acorn squash. It's topped with grilled tomatoes to give you a healthy dose of vitamin C and lycopene to start the day.

1 Preheat the oven to 200°C, gas mark 6. Fill a large saucepan with water and bring to the boil. Add the cubed potatoes and squash and cook for about 5 minutes until beginning to soften at the edges. Drain thoroughly and then spread out on a chopping board to cool slightly. Pat lightly with kitchen towel to dry.

2 Meanwhile, heat the oil in a small frying pan over low heat and fry the onion and garlic for 10 minutes until softened. Add the caraway seeds and paprika and cook for another 5 minutes. Stir in the potatoes and squash.

3 Tip the contents of the frying pan onto a baking tray and spread the vegetables out. Transfer to the top of the oven and bake for 35–45 minutes until golden brown.

4 About 10 minutes before the vegetables are done, heat the grill to medium-high. Cut the tomatoes in half around the middle. Mix the breadcrumbs and Parmesan together. Place the tomatoes, cut side up, in the grill pan and top with the breadcrumb mixture. Grill for about 10 minutes until the topping is golden and the tomatoes are soft.

5 To serve, divide the cooked vegetables between individual plates and, using a biscuit cutter or ring mould, form into neat rounds. Top each one with a tomato half and sprinkle with the parsley.

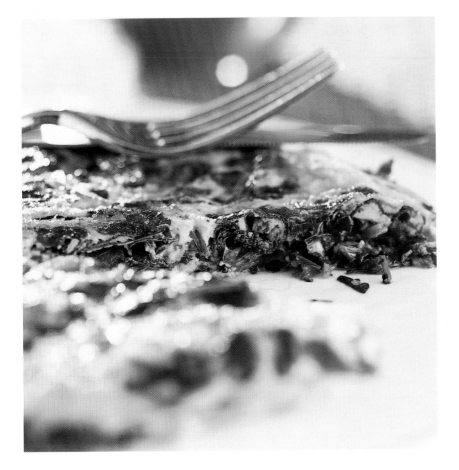

SPRINGTIME HERB FRITTATA

An open Spanish-style omelette packed with the superior flavour of fresh herbs. Use more sage for its oestrogen-mimicking ability to address hot flushes and night sweats.

1 Wash the herbs and remove any tough stalks. Roughly chop up all the leaves with the exception of any sage, leave these whole. Break the eggs into a bowl and beat with the milk and pepper.

2 Melt the butter in a small frying pan over medium-low heat until the butter is foaming – you need enough butter to finely coat the bottom of the pan. Add the herbs and cook for a few seconds. If using sage, cook the leaves for 5 minutes before adding the rest of the herbs.

3 Pour the beaten egg mixture into the pan and cook until the underside of the frittata is browned. Slide the frittata onto a plate and then invert the plate over the frying pan to turn the frittata into the pan and cook the underside. When the underside has browned, remove the frittata from the pan and leave to cool slightly before serving, cut into wedges.

50–75 g fresh herbs (use a mixture, such as basil, marjoram, sage, rocket, fennel, chervil, sorrel and celery leaves)

3 eggs

25 ml milk

½ teaspoon freshly ground black pepper

10–20 g butter

Serves 1–2

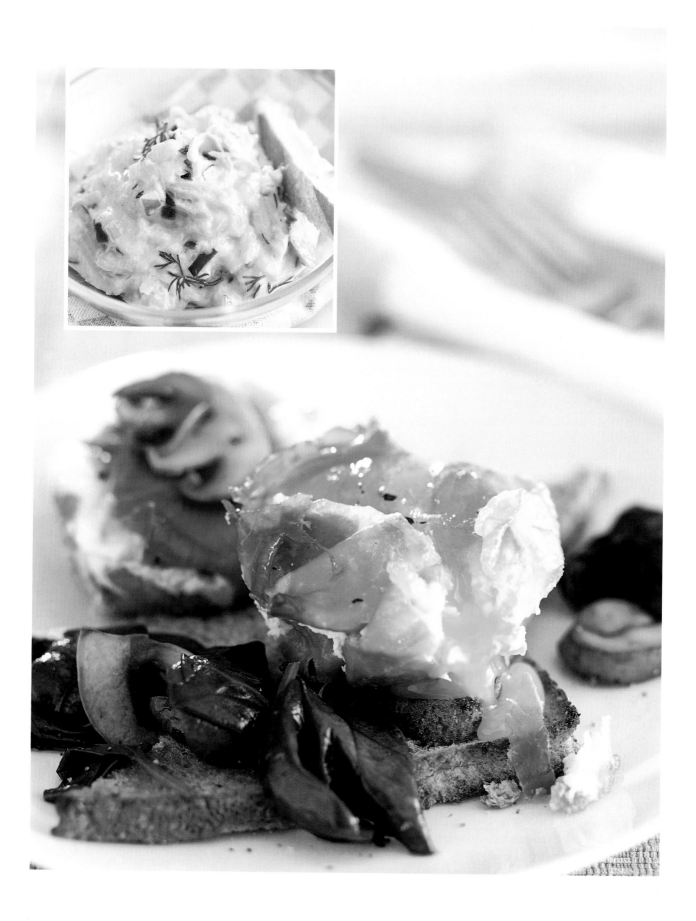

Baked Eggs & Mushrooms in Ham Crisps

An interesting alternative to bacon and eggs, this dish contains less fat than the traditional fry-up. It makes a substantial, well-balanced breakfast – ideal for high days and holidays.

1 Preheat the oven to 200°C, gas mark 6. Lightly grease inside and around the tops of 8 cups of a muffin tin with some oil. Place a cast-iron skillet or heavy-based frying pan over medium heat. When the pan is hot, dry fry the mushrooms for 10 minutes until they darken, release their juices and then re-absorb them. Cool slightly, then mix with the yogurt and pepper.

2 Place one slice of ham in each of the muffin cups, pressing it in, to make a well. Allow the ham to overlap the edges. Set aside 3 spoonfuls of mushroom mixture as garnish, then use the rest to fill the ham-lined cups.

3 Break the eggs, one at a time, into a jug. Gently tip each egg into the cups, taking care the egg white doesn't run over the edges of the muffin tin.

4 Bake for 10 minutes until the whites are set but the yolks are runny. Meanwhile, wash the spinach and, with water still clinging to the leaves, place in a saucepan over medium heat. Cook for a few minutes, stirring, until just wilted. Toast the bread. Carefully ease each Ham Crisp out of the muffin tin and serve at once with the toast and wilted spinach, garnished with the reserved mushrooms.

Rapeseed or sunflower oil, for greasing

5 large mushrooms, very finely sliced

1 tablespoon Greek yogurt

½ teaspoon freshly ground black pepper

8 slices very finely sliced Parma ham or pancetta

8 eggs

150 g baby spinach leaves

4 slices wholemeal bread

Serves 4

Creamy Scrambled Eggs with Smoked Trout

A filling start to the day, this is an ideal dish for a breakfast-time treat. Using low-fat cream cheese will reduce the calorific content.

1 Break the trout fillet up into small pieces. Cut the cream cheese into small pieces. Whisk the eggs in a large bowl until well blended. Stir in the trout, cream cheese, red onion and dill. Cut the ciabatta into thin strips and toast; keep warm.

2 Melt the butter in a cast-iron skillet or large non-stick frying pan over medium heat until the butter is foaming, do not allow it to brown.

3 Pour in the eggs and turn down the heat to low. Cook, stirring constantly, for 5 minutes until the mixture is lightly scrambled. Remove the pan from the heat and serve at once with the toasted ciabatta.

100 g smoked trout fillet

100 g firm cream cheese

8 eggs

½ red onion, finely chopped

½ teaspoon chopped fresh dill

Large knob of butter

Ciabatta bread, to serve

Serves 4

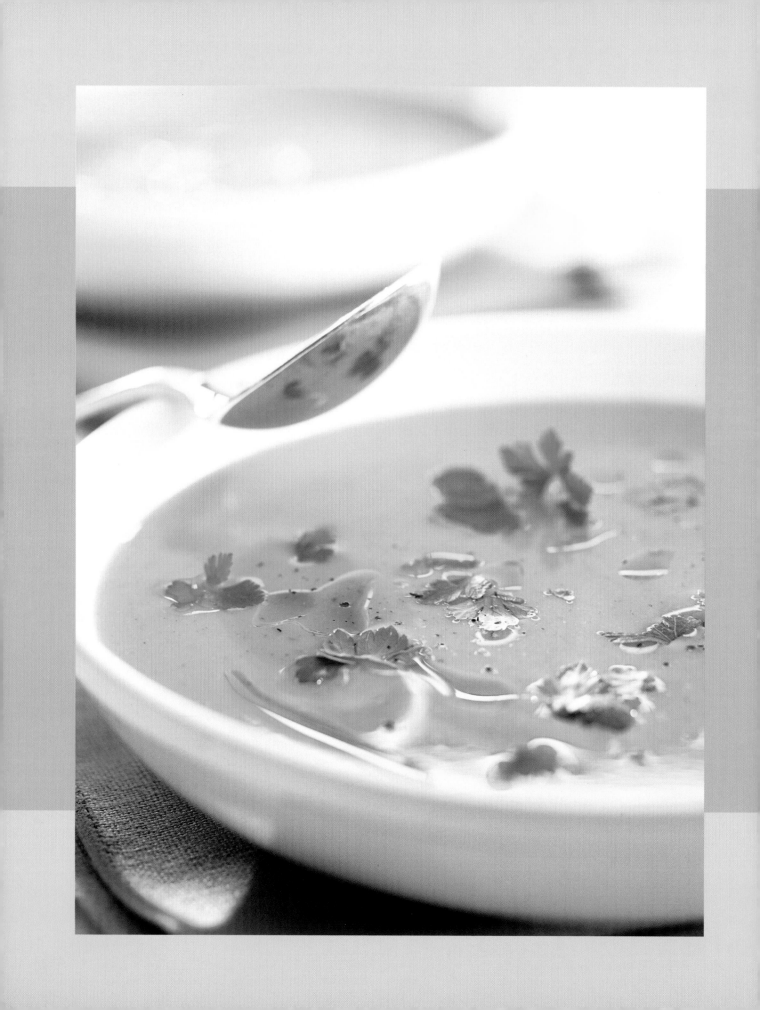

2
Soups & Starters

When you're planning a menu you want to get the best out of all the courses so look to this chapter for some wonderful and wholesome soups and starters that taste as good as they look.

CARROT & ORANGE SOUP

2 tablespoons olive oil

1 onion, finely chopped

500 g carrots, diced

750 ml vegetable stock

250 ml orange juice

2 teaspoons finely grated orange zest,
plus a few extra strips to garnish

Freshly ground black pepper, to serve

Serves 4

Eating carrots may help lower your risk of certain cancers and also helps with night vision. Fresh orange juice is a good source of vitamin C, which is essential for healthy skin and in building up the body's resistance to viruses.

1 Heat the oil in a large saucepan over medium heat and add the onion. Cook for 2–3 minutes until translucent. Add the carrots and cook for a further 5 minutes until slightly softened.

2 Pour the stock into the saucepan and raise the heat to medium-high. Bring to the boil then reduce the heat, cover and simmer for 30 minutes.

3 Allow the soup to cool slightly then process until smooth, using a food processor or blender and working in batches if necessary. Pour the soup back into the saucepan and stir in the orange juice and zest. Reheat gently and serve garnished with the extra zest and sprinkled with black pepper.

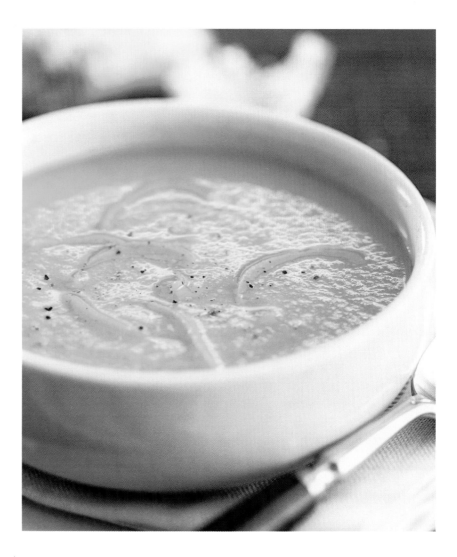

YELLOW CAULIFLOWER SOUP WITH CRUSTY CROUTONS

Made with milk, this is a high-calcium soup. Cauliflower is one of the crucifer vegetables, that may help reduce the risk of cancers.

1 Wash the cauliflower and separate it into small florets. Heat the oil in a large saucepan over low heat. Add the cumin and turmeric and cook for 3 minutes.

2 Add the cauliflower and spring onions and turn in the oil; sauté for a few minutes until just softened. Add the milk to the pan and raise the heat to medium-high. Bring the soup to a boil then reduce the heat to low and simmer, covered, for 30 minutes.

3 Meanwhile, make the croutons. Preheat the oven to 200°C, gas mark 6. Mix the Parmesan and oil together in a bowl and add the cubes of bread, turning them in the cheese mixture until well coated. Spread the coated bread out on a baking tray and transfer to the second shelf of the oven. Bake for 15 minutes until crisp and golden.

4 Using a food processor or blender, process the soup until smooth, working in batches if necessary. Season to taste and reheat gently to serve, sprinkled with the chives and accompanied by the croutons.

LEEK AND POTATO SOUP

This recipe works just as well using leeks and potatoes. Take two large baking potatoes and peel and dice them. Trim off the green part of two large leeks and roughly chop the remaining white parts; wash and drain thoroughly. Then just add the potatoes and leeks to the saucepan at step 2 instead of the cauliflower and spring onion.

---

1 medium cauliflower

1 tablespoon olive oil

1 teaspoon ground cumin

1 teaspoon turmeric

6 spring onions, white parts only, roughly chopped

750 ml milk

Salt and pepper, to taste

1 tablespoon chopped fresh chives

FOR THE CROUTONS

25 g Parmesan, freshly grated

5 tablespoons olive oil

100 g wholemeal bread, crusts removed and cut into 3 cm cubes

Serves 4

MUSHROOM SOUP WITH MISO

450 g mixed mushrooms, such as shitake, oyster, chestnut

6 spring onions

2 tablespoons olive oil

2 cloves garlic

2 tablespoons chopped fresh parsley

1 teaspoon miso paste

1.5 litres vegetable stock

2 slices wholemeal bread, crusts removed and cut into 1 cm cubes

125 ml unsweetened soya milk

2 tablespoons chopped fresh chives, to garnish

A few sage leaves, to garnish

Serves 6–8

You can make this highly flavoured soup with a variety of different mushrooms. The miso and soya milk are good sources of phytoestrogens, which may help reduce menopausal symptoms and heart disease.

1　Thinly slice the mushrooms and spring onions. Heat the oil in a large saucepan over low heat and add the spring onions; cook until softened. Stir in the garlic and parsley.

2　Mix the miso paste with a little water and stir it into the pan. Cook for 3 minutes more. Add the mushrooms and cook, covered, for 10 minutes.

3　Add the stock and bread and raise the heat until the soup comes to the boil. Then reduce the heat and simmer for 40 minutes.

4　Allow the soup to cool a little then process briefly, using a food processor or blender, so that the soup has a little texture and isn't completely smooth. Pour the soup back into the saucepan and add the soya milk. Reheat gently then serve at once, sprinkled with the chopped chives and sage leaves.

INGREDIENTS GUIDE

Miso is a paste made from fermented soy beans. It's very popular in Japanese cooking where it is used to flavour all sorts of soups, stews and sauces. If you can't find miso in the supermarket, then try a specialist Japanese or Oriental store or health-food shop.

If you can't get miso then you could use dashi, another popular Japanese ingredient, although the flavour of the soup will be different. Dashi is a clear light stock made from a type of seaweed called kombu and dried bonito (a fish similar to tuna). You can buy instant dashi in sachets. Simply make it up with hot water just as you would with any other stock powder and use it in place of the miso and vegetable stock.

EASY LENTIL SOUP

Lentils are a good source of soluble fibre and protein but are low in fat. They are broken down slowly by the body so can keep you full for a long time. The betacarotene in carrots converts to vitamin A, which strengthens the immune system.

1 Heat the oil in a large saucepan over medium-low heat and add the onions; cook for 2–5 minutes until soft. Add the lentils, carrots and stock.

2 Turn up the heat and bring the soup to a boil and then immediately reduce heat to low. Simmer, covered, for 45 minutes.

3 Stir in the lemon juice and allow the soup to cool slightly. Season to taste. Process half the soup, using a food processor or blender, until smooth. Stir the processed soup back into the rest of the soup and reheat gently to serve.

2 tablespoons olive oil

2 onions, finely chopped

350 g no-soak split red lentils

2 carrots, chopped

1.75 litres vegetable stock

Juice of 1 lemon

Freshly ground black pepper, to taste

Serves 6

PEA & BROCCOLI SOUP

Soup is an ideal way to get the most out of your cooked vegetables since the cooking liquid is part of the dish, instead of being discarded. Soya milk is used to add an extra boost of phytoestrogens – the vegetables already contain some.

1 Break up the broccoli into fairly small florets and chop the stalk. Heat the oil in a large saucepan over medium heat and fry the onions for about 5 minutes until translucent. Add the garlic and cook gently for another 5 minutes.

2 Add the stock and bring to a boil. Add the peas and return to the boil before adding the broccoli. Season to taste. Reduce the heat to low and simmer, covered, for 30 minutes.

3 Meanwhile, mix the olive oil and parsley together and set aside.

4 Using a food processor or blender, process the soup until smooth, working in batches if necessary. Stir in the soya milk and reheat gently, without allowing the soup to boil.

5 To serve, pour the soup into individual bowls and drizzle on the oil and parsley mixture.

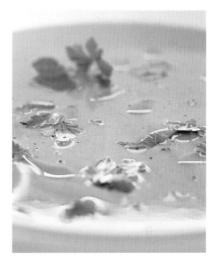

1 large head broccoli

3 tablespoons olive oil

3 onions, roughly chopped

1 clove garlic, crushed

2 litres vegetable stock

600 g frozen peas

Salt and pepper, to taste

2 tablespoons olive oil

1 tablespoon chopped fresh parsley

100 ml unsweetened soya milk

Serves 6–8

BARLEY BEAN SOUP

2 tablespoons olive oil

2 onions, roughly chopped

2 stalks celery, sliced

2 cloves garlic, finely sliced

1 teaspoon dried oregano

1 teaspoon dried marjoram

1 litre vegetable stock

100 g barley

225 g canned kidney beans

500 ml milk or unsweetened soya milk

2 teaspoons chopped fresh parsley

Freshly ground black pepper, to taste

Serves 6

Barley and kidney beans contain soluble fibre and so may help lower cholesterol and relieve constipation – all common problems after the menopause.

1 Heat the oil in a large saucepan over medium heat and add the onion, celery, garlic and dried herbs. Cook for 10 minutes until the vegetables are softened.

2 Pour in the stock and stir in the barley. Increase the heat to bring the soup to a boil, then reduce the heat to low, cover and simmer for 1 hour.

3 Drain and rinse the kidney beans then add them to the pan. Add the milk and parsley and season with pepper, to taste. Cook, uncovered, over low heat, for another 10 minutes until everything is hot; serve.

QUICK SCOTCH BROTH

You can adapt this recipe to make a simple version of the classic Scotch broth that's also an excellent way to use up left-over roast lamb. Peel 2 carrots and 2 baby turnips and cut into 2 cm cubes. Add them to the saucepan in step 1 with the onion, celery and garlic. Use a couple of teaspoons of dried thyme rather than oregano or marjoram and cook for 10 minutes. Add 1.5 litres stock – preferably lamb – and the barley and cook as in step 2. Trim any fat from the cooked lamb – you'll need at least 60 g per person – and cut into small pieces. Add to the pan at step 3 instead of the kidney beans and cook for another 20 minutes. Omit the milk and just sprinkle the parsley on the soup to serve.

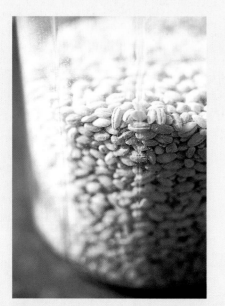

SCARLET SOUP

A vividly coloured soup, perfect for winter months, that's high in vitamins B and C and a good source of vegetable protein.

1 Heat the grill to its highest setting. Cut the pepper in half lengthways and remove the stalk, seeds and pith and discard. Grill the two halves, skin side up, until the skin is nicely charred. Allow to cool and then peel off the skin. Chop the flesh roughly; reserve.

2 Heat the oil in a large saucepan over medium heat and cook the onions and carrots for 5–7 minutes, until softened.

3 Add the red pepper, tomatoes, lentils, black pepper and stock and bring to a boil. Reduce the heat to low and simmer for 40 minutes.

4 Using a food processor or blender, process the soup until smooth, working in batches if necessary. Reheat gently, without allowing the soup to boil, and serve.

1 red pepper

2 tablespoons olive oil

2 onions, finely chopped

2 carrots, finely chopped

450 g canned chopped tomatoes

250 g red lentils

1 teaspoon freshly ground black pepper

2 litres vegetable stock

Serves 6–8

SMOKED TOFU CHOWDER

This is a great way to eat tofu – also known as soya bean curd and a great source of calcium and phytoestrogens. The tofu is liquidised and then used to thicken the soup.

1 Heat the oil in a large saucepan over medium heat and cook the onion and garlic, stirring occasionally, for 5–7 minutes until soft and translucent. Add the diced squash and courgette and cook for about 5 minutes more, stirring occasionally, until the vegetables are slightly softened. Add the stock and raise the heat to high. Bring to the boil then reduce the heat and simmer, covered, for 30 minutes.

2 Using a food processor or blender, process the soup in batches until smooth. Add the cubed tofu to the last batch and liquidise with the soup. Stir this back into the rest of the soup.

3 Stir in the sweetcorn and re-heat the soup gently. Add a few drops of fresh lemon juice and some black pepper, to taste. Serve sprinkled with the grated cheese, if liked.

1 tablespoon olive oil

1 onion, finely chopped

1 clove garlic, crushed

450 g butternut squash, peeled and diced

1 large courgette, diced

1 litre vegetable stock

220 g smoked tofu, drained and roughly cubed

200 g can sweetcorn, drained and rinsed

Freshly squeezed lemon juice, to taste

Freshly ground black pepper to taste

50 g Gouda, grated (optional)

Serves 4–6

MEDITERRANEAN FISH SOUP

2 tablespoons olive oil

2 onions, finely chopped

2 sticks celery, finely chopped

2 cloves garlic, crushed

¼ teaspoon smoked paprika

450 g canned chopped tomatoes

I litre fish stock

500 g fish, such as salmon, cod, haddock, sole, plaice, halibut or hake, all skin and bones removed

225 g raw prawns, shelled

Salt and pepper, to taste

Serves 4

A delicious soup – if you use salmon, it's high in the Omega 3 oils that help protect the heart and may help with joint problems. The tomatoes are rich in cancer-fighting lycopene.

1   Heat the oil in a large saucepan over low heat and cook the onion, celery, garlic and paprika gently for about 5 minutes until soft but not brown.

2   Add the tomatoes and stock and turn the heat up to high. Bring to the boil, add the fish and reduce the heat to low. Cover and simmer for 10 minutes.

3   Remove the lid and add the prawns. Cook, uncovered, for 5–10 minutes until the prawns are pink and all the fish is cooked through. Season to taste and serve.

FENNEL & RADICCHIO SALAD

2 fennel bulbs

I large head radicchio

50 g black olives

50 g walnut halves

2 canned anchovy fillets

100 ml olive oil

I tablespoon lemon juice

2 teaspoons finely chopped fresh thyme, plus a few sprigs to garnish

Serves 4

Fennel is a lovely anise-flavoured vegetable, with a crunchy texture. It requires little preparation either raw or cooked. The olives, walnuts and anchovies are rich in the heart-protecting Omega 3 and monosaturated oils.

1   Wash and trim the fennel and radicchio. Finely shred the fennel and tear the radicchio into even strips; transfer both to a large bowl.

2   Halve the olives lengthways and remove the stones. Add them to the bowl with the walnuts.

3   Finely chop the anchovies and place them in a jug with the oil, lemon juice and chopped thyme; whisk together. Pour on to the salad and toss well. Serve garnished with sprigs of fresh thyme.

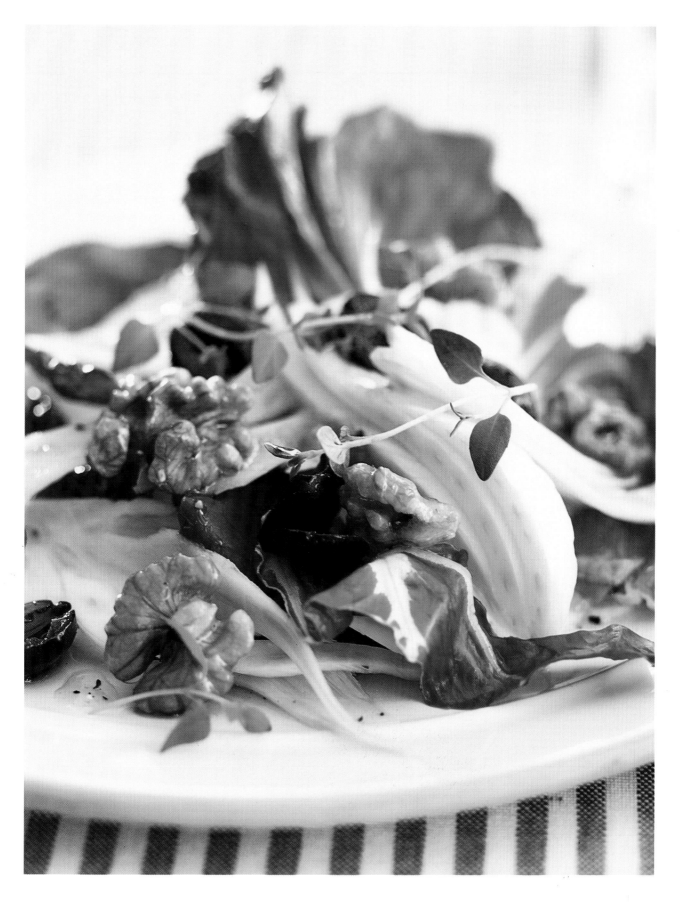

CHARRED NECTARINES

40 g pine nuts

4 nectarines, stoned and halved

100 g bag rocket leaves

4 tablespoons olive oil

4 teaspoons balsamic vinegar

Serves 4

This summer fruit appetiser is high in betacarotene, vitamin C and flavonoids, plant pigments that have anti-oxidant properties. Pine nuts are rich in essential fatty acids, which can help protect the heart.

1   Heat the grill to high. Place the pine nuts on a foil-lined baking tray and toast under the grill for a few seconds. Do not allow to burn.

2   Heat a cast-iron skillet or heavy-based frying pan until very hot. Place the nectarine halves flesh side down into the pan. Cook for 5–7 minutes until a crust begins to form on the flesh.

3   Divide the rocket leaves between individual serving plates. Drizzle the oil and then the vinegar over the leaves.

4   Place two nectarine halves on top of each plate and sprinkle with the toasted pine nuts. Serve while still warm.

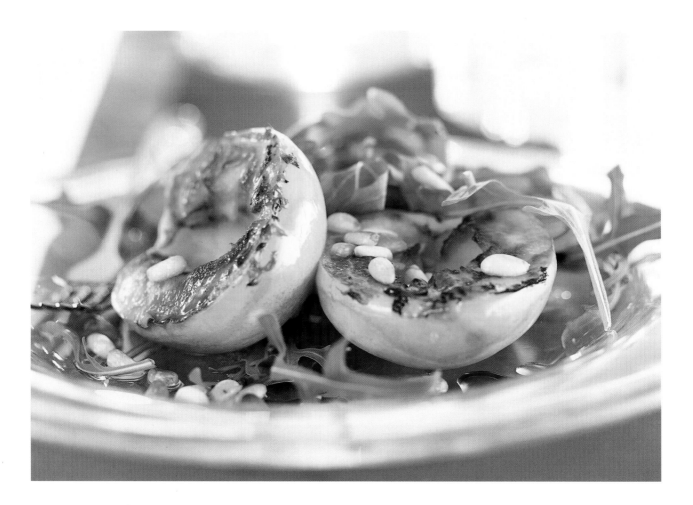

WATERCRESS & AVOCADO SALAD WITH PITTA BREAD & HUMOUS

Watercress and humous are both good sources of calcium. Avocados, although rich in oil, contain the more healthy monosaturated oils. Sunflower seeds are packed with Omega 3 oils and phytoestrogens.

1	To make the humous, place the chickpeas, tahini, olive oil and garlic in a food processor or blender and process until smooth. Add a few drops of the lemon juice to taste.
2	Wash, drain and dry the watercress thoroughly. Transfer to a large shallow serving dish. Cut the avocados in half and remove the stones. Remove the peel and cut lengthways into thin slices. Arrange over the watercress and sprinkle with sunflower seeds.
3	Whisk the walnut oil and remaining lemon juice together and season with pepper. Pour over the salad.
4	Toast the pitta breads until warm. Cut each one in half and open out to form a pocket. Fill with the humous and serve with the salad.

400 g can chickpeas, drained and rinsed

2 tablespoons tahini

1 tablespoon olive oil

4 cloves garlic, crushed

2 tablespoons freshly squeezed lemon juice

100 g watercress

2 avocados

60 g sunflower seeds

2 tablespoons walnut oil

Freshly ground black pepper, to taste

4 pitta breads

Serves 4

BEAN BURRITOS

This tasty starter or snack is based on the classic Mexican dish. It uses the plain, pancake-like tortillas that are then covered with a delicious bean filling and rolled up to eat. Beans are a good low-fat source of protein, calcium and soluble fibre.

1	Preheat the oven to 140°C, gas mark 1. Wrap the tortillas in tin foil and place in the oven to warm through.
2	Heat the oil in a large frying pan over medium and fry the spring onions for 2 minutes. Stir in the chilli powder and cook for a few seconds more.
3	Stir in the beans, stock and tomato purée. Raise the heat and bring to a boil. Reduce the heat to low and simmer, uncovered, for 10–15 minutes, stirring occasionally, until almost all the liquid has evaporated.
4	Using a potato masher, roughly mash the beans – you don't want to completely pulverise them, there should be some bits of bean left in the mixture. Stir in the chopped parsley.
5	Take a tortilla and spread with an eighth of the bean mixture. Add a couple of spoonfuls of yogurt and then roll up the tortilla. Repeat with the remaining tortillas, bean mixture and yogurt and serve at once.

8 small ready-made tortillas

1 tablespoon olive oil

2 large spring onions, chopped

¼ teaspoon chilli powder

400 g can kidney beans or borlotti beans, drained and rinsed

400 g can chickpeas or cannellini beans, drained and rinsed

125 ml vegetable stock

1 teaspoon tomato purée

2 tablespoons finely chopped fresh parsley

80–100 g plain Greek yogurt

Serves 4

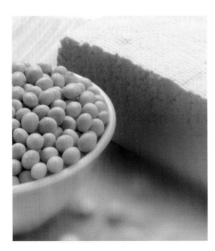

WARM SALAD WITH TOFU PARMESAN

Tofu, or soya bean curd, is an excellent source of calcium and plant oestrogens – also known as phytoestrogens. Try this version of a salade tiede, *which uses crispy coated tofu and griddled aubergine and courgette.*

175 g firm tofu

25 g breadcrumbs

3 tablespoons grated Parmesan cheese

1 teaspoon dried oregano

½ teaspoon freshly ground black pepper

1 egg, beaten

2–4 tablespoons olive oil

1 courgette

1 aubergine

100 g bag mixed salad leaves

1 tablespoon flax oil

2 teaspoons balsamic vinegar

1 teaspoon sesame seeds

Serves 4

1 Take the tofu out of its packaging, draining off any liquid. Place the tofu on top of three sheets of kitchen towel and pat lightly. When the kitchen towel is soaked through, repeat with some fresh sheets. Repeat the process until the tofu is quite dry. Cut the tofu into 2 cm thick slices.

2 Mix the breadcrumbs, Parmesan, oregano and black pepper together in a small bowl. Dip the dried slices of tofu into the beaten egg and then immediately into the breadcrumb mixture, and place on a plate.

3 Heat 2 tablespoons olive oil in a frying pan over medium-high heat and fry the coated tofu, in batches, until crisp on one side. Turn and cook the other side until crisp. Keep the cooked tofu warm.

4 Cut the courgette and aubergine diagonally into thin slices. Brush each slice on both sides with olive oil. Place a griddle pan over a high heat and when the pan is hot add the vegetables. Cook in batches until nicely charred and soft. Keep the cooked vegetables warm.

5 To assemble the salad, spread the leaves over a large shallow serving bowl and drizzle with the flax oil and balsamic vinegar. Arrange the griddled vegetables over the leaves and top with the tofu. Sprinkle on the sesame seeds. Toss everything together to serve.

TOFU MAYONNAISE OPEN SANDWICH

The phytoestrogens in tofu can help ease hot flushes and other symptoms of the menopause. Use the tofu mayonnaise as an appetiser with a green salad or as a sandwich filling with cress.

1 Take the tofu out of its packaging, draining off any liquid. Place the tofu on top of three sheets of kitchen towel and pat lightly. When the kitchen towel is soaked through, repeat with some fresh sheets. Repeat the process until the tofu is quite dry. Grate it into a bowl.

2 Mix together the mayonnaise, mustard, turmeric, dill, parsley and black pepper in a separate bowl. Stir in the spring onions and celery.

3 Fold the grated tofu into the mayonnaise mixture and chill for at least 1 hour to let the mixture firm up and the flavours develop.

4 To serve, place a slice of rye bread on each plate and top each slice with the tofu mayonnaise. Garnish with the extra sprigs of dill.

450 g firm tofu

4 tablespoons mayonnaise

2 teaspoons Dijon mustard

¼ teaspoon turmeric

1 tablespoon chopped fresh dill, plus a few extra sprigs to garnish

1 tablespoon finely chopped fresh parsley

1 teaspoon freshly ground black pepper

3 spring onions, finely chopped

1 stalk celery, finely chopped

4 thick slices rye bread

Serves 4

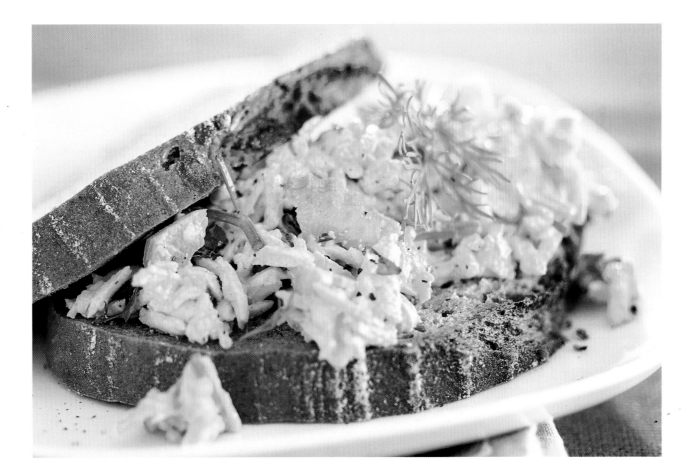

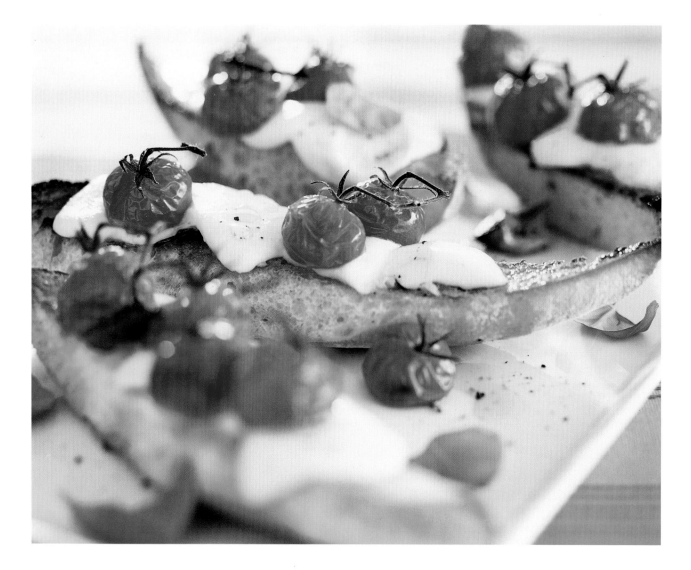

MOZZARELLA CIABATTA BITES

A modern version of a cheese and tomato sandwich – almost a 'cheat's pizza'. The mozzarella is a good source of calcium and contains about a third less fat than hard cheese.

250 g vine-ripened cherry tomatoes

2 small ciabatta loaves

3 tablespoons olive oil

1 clove garlic, crushed

8 fresh basil leaves, chopped

2 x 150 g packs mozzarella, drained and sliced

Serves 4

1 Heat the oven to 180°C, gas mark 5. Place the tomatoes on a baking tray and roast for 30 minutes until they soften or begin to brown slightly.

2 Meanwhile, cut the ciabatta loaves in half lengthways then cut each piece in half lengthways again; toast. Mix the oil, garlic and basil in a bowl and brush this on one side of each piece of toast, reserving a few drops.

3 Heat the grill to high. Lay out the toast, oil-brushed side up, on the grill pan and top with the mozzarella and roasted tomatoes. Drizzle with the reserved oil mixture. Grill for a few seconds, until the cheese begins to melt slightly and everything is warmed through.

GORGONZOLA, WATERCRESS & FIG SALAD

Watercress is rich in vitamins A and C and contains potassium and calcium. The walnuts and figs provide a good source of fibre in this dish.

1 Heat the grill to high and spread the walnuts over a foil-lined baking tray. Toast under grill for a moment, until a nutty smell begins to rise; cool.

2 Wash, drain and thoroughly dry the watercress. Scatter over a large plate or shallow serving dish.

3 Whisk the oil, vinegar and mayonnaise together to make the dressing. Crumble the cheese over the watercress and then top with the figs. Pour over the dressing and serve, sprinkled with the walnuts.

50 g chopped walnuts

200 g watercress

1 tablespoon olive oil

1 tablespoon cider vinegar

1 tablespoon mayonnaise

150 g Gorgonzola

4 ripe figs, quartered

Serves 4

GOAT'S CHEESE WITH BABY SPINACH & OLIVES

Goat's cheese is a flavoursome alternative to cow's milk cheese and is lower in fat. This dish contains calcium, phosphorous and vitamin D, which combine as good bone-builders.

1 Cut the cheeses in half, widthways, leaving on the rind. Dip the non-rind side of each piece in the beaten eggs and then in the flour, ensuring they are well coated.

2 Heat a cast iron skillet or heavy-based frying pan over high heat. Place the pieces of cheese floured-side down in the hot pan. Turn the heat down to medium-high and cook for 7–10 minutes, without moving the cheese, until they begin to ooze slightly. The underside of the cheese should be crusty and golden.

3 Divide the spinach between four serving plates. Sprinkle on the chives and olives. Turn the cheese, fried side up, on to the plates and serve accompanied by chutney.

2 rounds of mild goat's cheese

2 eggs, beaten

2 tablespoons flour

100 g baby spinach

2 tablespoons chopped fresh chives

50 g black olives, pitted

2 tablespoons any fruit chutney, to serve

Serves 4

SALMON CAKE HORS D'OEUVRES

500 ml fish stock

450 g salmon fillet, skin removed

I egg white, beaten

3 tablespoons plain flour

I teaspoon creamed horseradish sauce

3 tablespoons chopped fresh parsley

Rapeseed or sunflower oil, to shallow fry

FOR THE DIPPING SAUCE

100 ml lime juice

100 ml soy sauce

2 tablespoons soft light brown sugar

Makes about 10 small fish cakes

These little fish cakes make a tasty salmon starter – a great way to eat more of this healthy oily fish. This recipe cooks the fish from scratch but you could use left-over cooked salmon.

1 Pour the stock into a large saucepan or sauté pan, place over medium-high heat and bring to a boil. Put the salmon in the stock. When the stock has returned to the boil, reduce the heat to low and cover. Simmer for 15 minutes until the fish flakes easily when tested with the point of a knife. Drain and set aside to cool.

2 When cool, flake the salmon into a bowl. Add the beaten egg white, flour, horseradish sauce and parsley. Mix together well. Wet your hands and form the mixture into small cakes 5–6 cm in diameter, flattening each one slightly with the palm of your hand. Chill the salmon cakes for 30 minutes in the fridge.

3 Pour enough oil into a large frying pan to cover the bottom and place over medium-high heat. When the oil is hot, fry the salmon cakes for about 3 minutes on each side until they are crispy, working in batches. Drain on kitchen towel.

4 To make the dipping sauce, whisk the lime juice, soy sauce and brown sugar together, making sure the sugar has dissolved. Serve the salmon cakes warm or cold, accompanied by the dipping sauce.

LEMONY TARTARE DIPPING SAUCE

Tartare sauce is a traditional accompaniment to fish. You can make a creamy alternative to the dipping sauce that uses typical tartare flavours and a hint of lemon. Beat together 7 tablespoons of good quality mayonnaise with 3 tablespoons crème fraîche. Stir in 1 teaspoon grated lemon zest, 1 tablespoon chopped capers and 1 tablespoon chopped gherkins or cornichons. This should make about 180 ml of dipping sauce.

SMOKED MACKEREL APPETISER

Make the most of smoked mackerel fillets with this tasty dish. Mackerel is an oily fish and so a good source of vitamin D and essential Omega 3 oils for heart health. Serve with sliced and toasted rye bread.

1   Remove the skin from the mackerel and flake the flesh, using two forks; transfer to a bowl. Mash the eggs with the horseradish and add to the bowl with the celery; mix together well.

2   Gradually beat the lemon juice into the mixture until it has a pâté-like consistency. Transfer to a serving dish and sprinkle with the ground peppercorns to garnish, if liked. Cover and chill for at least 2 hours before serving.

300 g smoked mackerel

2 hard boiled eggs

I tablespoon creamed horseradish sauce

I celery stalk, very finely chopped

Juice of ½ lemon

Ground red and green peppercorns to garnish (optional)

Serves 6

CHICKEN LIVER ANTIPASTI

Chicken livers are an excellent source of the B vitamins as well as iron and zinc. Although rich in cholesterol, this is not a problem if the rest of the diet is low in saturated fats.

1   Cut the lemon into slices. Put them and 100 ml water in a small pan over high heat and bring to a boil. When the water comes to a boil add the chicken livers and reduce to medium heat; cook for 2 minutes. Drain thoroughly and cool slightly before chopping them roughly.

2   Heat the oil in a heavy-based frying pan over medium-low heat and fry the celery and onion for about 5 minutes until soft. Add the parsley and sage and cook for another 10 minutes, stirring regularly.

3   Add the chicken livers and 50 ml stock. Cook for 5 minutes, stirring, adding a little extra stock if the pan starts to look dry. Stir in the anchovies and butter and cook for another 5 minutes over a gentle heat. Place the whole mixture in a bowl and cool. Chill for at least 2 hours.

4   When you're ready to serve, preheat the oven to 180°C, gas mark 4 and take the chicken liver mixture out of the fridge to bring it to room temperature. Cut the bread into 2 cm thick slices and lay on a baking tray. Bake for 10 minutes, turning the bread halfway through the cooking time. Take the bread out of the oven and top each slice with the chicken liver mixture. Serve garnished with sage and parsley leaves.

½ lemon

200 g chicken livers, trimmed

2 tablespoons olive oil

I stick celery, thinly sliced

I onion, chopped

I tablespoon finely chopped fresh parsley

3 fresh sage leaves, finely chopped

50–75 ml vegetable stock

2 canned anchovy fillets, chopped

15 g butter

½ baguette or I ciabatta loaf

Parsley and sage leaves, to garnish

Serves 4–6

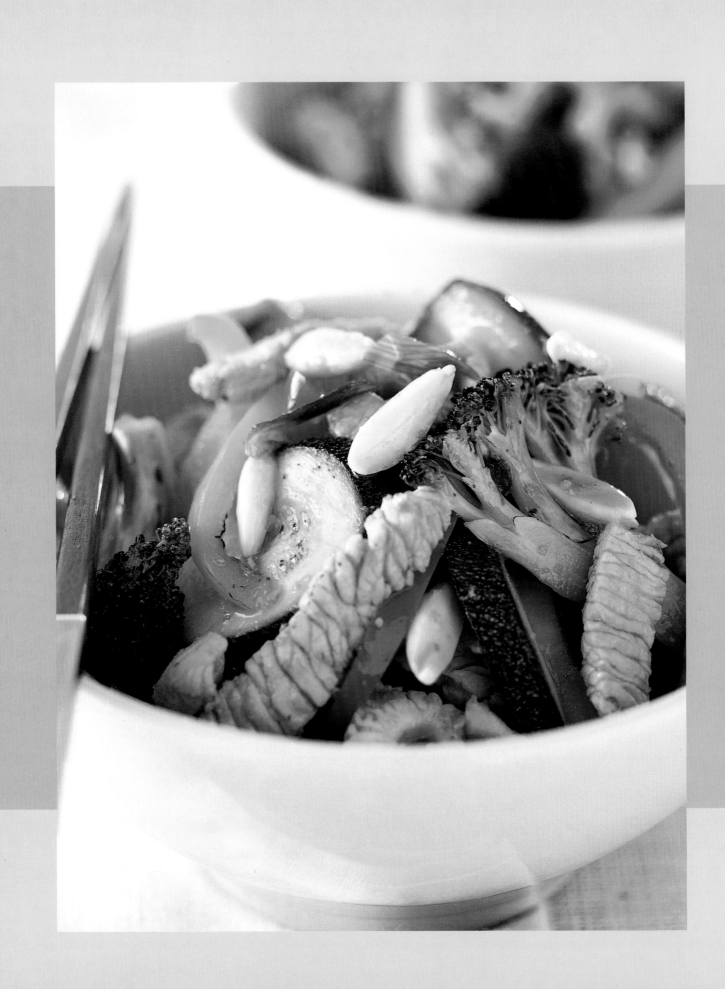

3
Light Lunches

When you want a light meal, whatever the time of day, you want something that's nutritious as well as delicious. This chapter offers you plenty of both tasty and healthy options.

FETA CHEESE PARCELS

20 g butter, melted

2 x 225 g packs feta cheese

1 tablespoon chopped fresh chives

6 fresh sage leaves, chopped

1 teaspoon freshly ground black pepper

225–275 g filo pastry

Serves 4

This is an ideal recipe if you want to avoid cow's milk cheese, yet still want a calcium-rich dish – feta is a goat's milk cheese. It also makes a very attractive meal – the filo is wrapped around the filling to form neat little parcels.

1 Preheat the oven to 200°C, gas mark 6. Brush a baking tray with some of the melted butter. Place the cheese in a bowl and mash with a fork. Add the chopped chives, sage and pepper and mix well.

2 Lay out one sheet of filo pastry and brush the sheet with melted butter. Lay another sheet on top and trim both to an 18 cm square. Brush the edges with more melted butter.

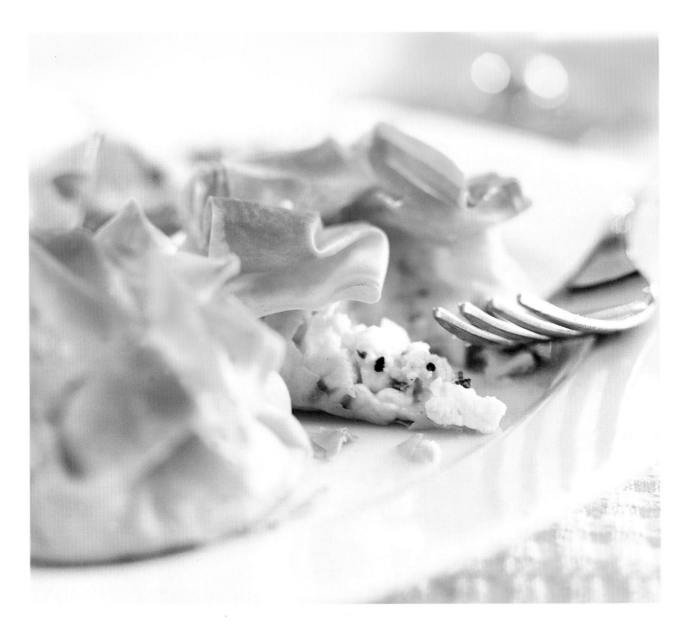

3   Place one eighth of the cheese mixture in the middle of the filo. Draw up the edges of the pastry around the cheese and scrunch up at the top to form a little bundle. Repeat with the remaining sheets of filo and cheese mixture to make seven more parcels.

4   Transfer the filo parcels to the greased baking tray and bake in the centre of the oven for 15 minutes, until crisp and golden brown. Allow to cool slightly before serving.

BROCCOLI, BROAD BEAN & FETA SALAD

This fresh and delicious summer lunch dish is rich in calcium, found in the broccoli, cheese and sesame seeds. The recipe uses feta cheese but you could substitute mozzarella.

200 g shelled broad beans
150 g broccoli florets
200 g feta cheese, cubed
2 cloves garlic, crushed
1 teaspoon Dijon mustard
4 teaspoons olive oil
1 teaspoon balsamic vinegar
Freshly ground black pepper, to taste
Sesame seeds, to serve
Serves 4

1   Fill a medium-sized saucepan with water and bring to the boil. Add the broad beans and cook on high for about 7 minutes. Drain and leave to cool for a few minutes. Cook the broccoli in the same way for 3 minutes. Drain and reserve.

2   Take the cooled beans and rub each one gently between your fingers to remove the tough, grey-green outer skin. Turn into a serving bowl and add the broccoli and feta cheese. Stir to combine.

3   To make the dressing, whisk the garlic, mustard, olive oil and vinegar together in a bowl or jug; season with pepper to taste. Just before serving, pour the dressing over the salad and sprinkle with some sesame seeds.

CHICKPEAS & SPINACH WITH GARLIC RICE

A Lebanese-style dish that can also be used as an accompaniment to roast meats. Serve the chickpeas warm, rather than hot, so flavours have a chance to blend.

2 teaspoons olive oil

2 cloves garlic, crushed

200 g basmati rice

1 onion, finely chopped

2 x 400 g cans chickpeas

4 tablespoons tomato purée

Pinch of cayenne pepper

Juice of 1 lemon

Freshly ground black pepper, to taste

200 g spinach, thoroughly washed

Serves 4

1. Heat 1 teaspoon olive oil in a large saucepan over medium heat and gently fry the garlic for about a minute. Add the rice and turn in the oil before adding 500 ml water. Bring to the boil then reduce the heat to low and simmer, covered, for 15–20 minutes until the grains of rice are tender.

2. Heat the remaining olive oil in a medium-sized saucepan and sauté the onion until soft. Stir in the undrained chickpeas. Bring to a boil and then add the tomato purée, cayenne, lemon juice and season to taste. Simmer uncovered for 10–15 minutes.

3. Add the spinach and stir into the chickpea mixture until it has completely wilted. Take the pan off the heat and set aside for a few minutes to cool very slightly before serving with the rice.

PESTO PARMESAN MUSHROOMS

Look for mushrooms that have deep cups so they can take as much of the tasty filling as possible. These make a delicious light lunch served with crusty bread.

40 g fresh basil

1 clove garlic, crushed

3 tablespoons pine nuts

75 g freshly grated Parmesan cheese

100 ml olive oil

8 large flat mushrooms

2 slices day-old bread, made into breadcrumbs

50 g chopped walnuts

Freshly ground black pepper, to taste

Serves 4

1. Preheat the oven to 180°C, gas mark 5. To make the pesto, place the basil, garlic and 2 tablespoons pine nuts in a food processor and process for a few seconds until everything is finely chopped. Add 50 g of the grated Parmesan and process for a few seconds more. Add the oil in a gentle stream while the motor is still running. Set the pesto aside.

2. Remove the stalks from the mushrooms and chop the stalks finely; set aside. Lay the whole mushrooms on a baking tray and put a spoonful of pesto in each cap. Mix the breadcrumbs with the chopped mushroom stalks and walnuts, season with pepper to taste. Divide the mixture between the mushrooms and use to top the pesto.

3. Sprinkle the remaining Parmesan cheese over the breadcrumb mixture. Sprinkle with the remaining pine nuts and bake in the middle of the oven for 10 minutes until the pine nuts turn a golden brown.

YELLOW PEPPERS WITH TURMERIC CAULIFLOWER & PARMESAN

An all-round bright and cheerful dish, with betacarotene from the pepper and anti-oxidants in the cauliflower, which makes an interesting alternative to cauliflower cheese.

1 Preheat the oven to 200°C, gas mark 6. Cut the peppers in half lengthways and remove the seeds, pith and stalk. Brush with olive oil and place on a baking tray. Bake on the top shelf for 20 minutes.

2 Meanwhile, break the cauliflower into very small florets. Fill a medium saucepan with water and place over high heat. Bring to a boil and add the cauliflower. Cook on a rapid boil for no more than 3 minutes then drain thoroughly and set aside.

3 Melt the butter in a saucepan over a low heat until it begins to foam. Add the onion and turmeric and cook for 10 minutes until the onion softens. Mix the cooked cauliflower in with the onion and turmeric.

4 Heat the grill to the highest setting. Fill each pepper half with some cauliflower mixture and sprinkle each one with Parmesan. Place under the grill for a few seconds until the cheese begins to melt.

4 yellow peppers

Olive oil, for brushing

1 cauliflower

A knob of butter

1 large onion, finely chopped

1 teaspoon ground turmeric

50 g Parmesan cheese, grated

Serves 4

GREEN PEPPER WITH BROCCOLI AND BLUE CHEESE

Use green peppers and prepare and bake them as above. Take a head of broccoli and cut it into small florets. Cook for 3–5 minutes until just tender. Finely chop 4 spring onions and sweat in a little butter over low heat until softened. Mix the spring onions with the cooked broccoli and season with a little freshly ground black pepper. Use the broccoli mixture to fill the green pepper halves. Crumble 80 g blue cheese and sprinkle over the top of the peppers. Grill until the cheese begins to melt.

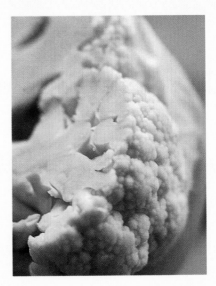

PRAWN PASTA

500 g fusilli or linguine

I tablespoon olive oil

I large onion, finely chopped

2 cloves garlic, crushed

2 tablespoons passata or sieved tomatoes

375 ml vegetable stock

225 g large raw prawns, shelled

3 tablespoons chopped fresh parsley

A few snipped chives, to garnish

Serves 4

This is a tasty way with seafood and pasta that creates a light but filling dish. Prawns are low in fat but rich in protein and so make an excellent occasional treat.

1 Fill a large saucepan with salted water and bring to the boil. Add the pasta and cook at a rolling boil for 10–15 minutes.

2 Meanwhile, heat the oil in a frying pan over medium heat and cook the onion and garlic for 5 minutes until softened. Add the passata and cook for a few seconds, stirring, then add the stock and bring to the boil. Add the prawns and reduce to a simmer. Cook for 5–10 minutes, until the prawns are pink and cooked through.

3 Stir the fresh parsley into the sauce. Drain the cooked pasta and combine with the prawn sauce. Garnish with the chives and serve at once.

SALMON CAKES

2 x 225 g cans salmon

I onion, grated

100–120 g matzo meal

I teaspoon freshly ground black pepper

I egg, beaten

Rapeseed or sunflower oil, for frying

Serves 4

Delicious hot or cold, serve these light fishcakes with thinly sliced cucumber and a dollop of mayonnaise on the side. If you can't get matzo meal use very fine breadcrumbs instead.

1 Drain the salmon but retain the liquid from one can. Mix the salmon, retained liquid, onion, 100 g matzo meal, pepper and the beaten egg together in a bowl. Shape the mixture into 5–7cm rounds. If the consistency isn't firm enough, add little more of the matzo meal.

2 Pour enough oil into a frying pan to come 1 cm up the sides. Heat until very hot. Add the fishcakes and fry, in batches, for 3–4 minutes on each side until they turn crispy. Drain on some paper towel then serve at once.

HOME-MADE GARLIC MAYONNAISE

These fish cakes are particularly good with mayonnaise and it is quite easy to make your own. Break an egg into a food processor and add 4 crushed garlic cloves and ¼ teaspoon coarse salt; process until everything is blended. With the motor running, pour 150 ml olive oil into the processor, a little at a time. With the motor still running, add 150 ml rapeseed oil in a gentle stream. Season with freshly ground black pepper to taste. This makes about 350 ml of mayonnaise.

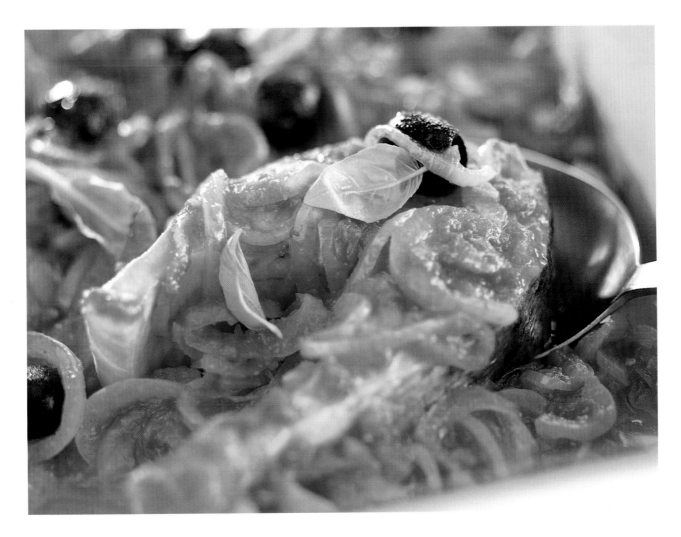

Mediterranean Fish

This recipe uses salmon but you could substitute another kind of thick fish steak such as hake or halibut. Serve it with plain new potatoes, or chips for a special treat.

1 Preheat the oven to 220°C, gas mark 7. Heat the oil in a medium-sized frying pan over medium heat and cook the onion and garlic for 2–5 minutes until translucent. Pour in the wine and let it bubble up.

2 Add the tomatoes and olives to the pan; add the sugar and season to taste. Cook for 10–15 minutes over low heat until the sauce has reduced slightly.

3 Place the salmon in a small non-metallic ovenproof dish, just big enough to take the steaks. Cover with the sauce and bake, uncovered, for 15–20 minutes until the fish is cooked through but hasn't dried out. Serve garnished with a few fresh basil leaves.

1 tablespoon olive oil

2 onions, finely sliced

2 cloves garlic, crushed

100 ml white wine

400 g can chopped tomatoes

50 g black olives, pitted and chopped

Pinch of sugar

Salt and pepper, to taste

4 salmon steaks

A few fresh basil leaves, to garnish

Serves 4

GRILLED HERRINGS WITH ORANGE SALSA

This colourful fish dish, high in B vitamins and Omega 3 oils, is served with a healthy flavoursome salsa that's packed with cancer-fighting phyto-chemicals.

70 g pine nuts

4 filleted herrings

I tablespoon olive oil

Salt and pepper, to taste

FOR THE SALSA

2 oranges

I yellow or orange pepper, diced

I red onion, chopped

5 fresh sage or mint leaves, chopped

Serves 4

1 Heat the grill to high. Line a baking tray with foil and sprinkle on the pine nuts. Toast under the grill for about 30 seconds until golden; set aside.

2 Open the herrings out flat and place, flesh-side down, on the foil-lined tray. Brush with the olive oil and season. Grill for 3–4 minutes until the fish is cooked through. Season to taste.

3 Meanwhile, make the salsa. Peel the orange and remove the pith. Chop the flesh and transfer to a bowl with any juices released during chopping. Stir in the pepper, onion and sage or mint.

4 Serve the cooked fish covered with a little salsa and sprinkled with the toasted pine nuts.

EASTERN SOLE

The simplest of fish dishes, very low in fat but full of aromatic seasoning. Sesame seeds contain bone-protecting calcium as well as essential fatty acids that can help protect against heart disease.

4 sole fillets

I teaspoon paprika

100 ml white wine

2 teaspoons soy sauce

3 teaspoons sesame seeds

Serves 4

1 Mix the paprika, wine and soy sauce together to make the marinade. Place the fish in a shallow non-metallic dish and pour on the marinade. Cover and set aside for at least 30 minutes.

2 Meanwhile, heat the grill to its highest setting. Line a baking tray with foil and spread out the sesame seeds. Toast for about 30 seconds under the grill until golden; set aside.

4 Place the fish on the baking tray skin side up and grill for 3–4 minutes, depending on the thickness of the fish. Turn, cover with a couple of teaspoons of the marinade and grill for another 3 minutes. Serve, sprinkled with the toasted sesame seeds.

SLIGHTLY SPICY FISH GOUJONS

A slightly spicy coating puts some pep into these fish goujons – you can omit the curry powder if you're particularly troubled by hot flushes. Paprika is a mild, sweet spice and a good way to add a little gentle 'heat' to this dish.

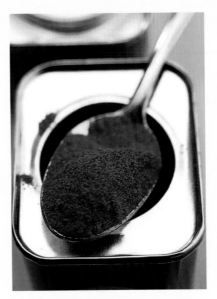

1 Cut the fish into 2–3 cm wide strips. Place in a shallow non-metallic dish and cover with the lime juice. Cover and set aside for 30 minutes.

2 Mix the cumin, curry powder, paprika and flour together in a bowl. Dip each piece of fish in the mixture until well coated.

3 Pour enough oil into a cast-iron skillet or large frying pan to come 1 cm up the sides. Heat until very hot. Fry the goujons, in batches, over high heat for 3 minutes or until they become crisp and golden. Drain on paper towel and serve at once.

1 kg skinned cod fillet
Juice of 1 lime
2 teaspoons ground cumin
2 teaspoons mild curry powder
1 teaspoon paprika
150 g plain flour
Rapeseed or sunflower oil, for frying
Serves 4

PEANUT SAUCE

To make a satay-inspired sauce to go with these goujons, put 115 g smooth unsweetened peanut butter in a food processor or blender and add 1 crushed garlic clove. Process together for a few seconds then add 1 tablespoon soy sauce, 5 tablespoons coconut milk, 1 teaspoon lime juice and 1 teaspoon runny honey and process again.

TOMATO SAUCE

For a tomato dipping sauce with a hint of spice, take 800 g of ripe tomatoes and skin and deseed them before dicing the flesh. Heat 1 tablespoon rapeseed or sunflower oil in a frying pan over medium heat and add 2 finely chopped shallots, 1 crushed garlic clove and a peeled and grated 2 cm piece of fresh ginger root. Fry gently for about 5 minutes until the shallot is translucent. Stir in 1 teaspoon ground cumin and ½ teaspoon ground fenugreek and cook for about 1 minute more. Stir in the tomatoes, turn the heat to low and cook gently for 5–8 minutes, stirring occasionally, until the tomatoes are softened. Allow to cool then transfer to a food processor or blender and purée. Press through a sieve for a smooth sauce.

WARM MACKEREL SALAD WITH POTATOES & OLIVES

500 g new potatoes

500 g smoked mackerel fillets

50 g green olives, pitted

2 tablespoons chopped fresh parsley

2 canned anchovy fillets, finely chopped

3 tablespoons olive oil

1 tablespoon oil from the can of anchovies

2 tablespoons cider vinegar

1 teaspoon Dijon mustard

Freshly ground black pepper, to taste

4 hard-boiled eggs

Serves 4

This substantial salad makes an ideal lunch dish. Mackerel is an oily fish that helps protects the heart and which may ease arthritis and combat depression.

1 Bring a large pan of water to the boil and cook the potatoes for 20 minutes until tender. Drain and cut into chunks when cool enough to handle. Set aside and keep warm.

2 Meanwhile, flake the smoked mackerel into a serving dish or bowl. Stir in the olives, parsley and anchovies.

3 To make the dressing, beat the olive oil, oil from the anchovies, vinegar and mustard together in a jug; season with pepper to taste. Mix the potatoes with the mackerel in the serving dish.

4 Peel the hard-boiled eggs and cut into quarters. Fold them in with the potatoes and mackerel and pour on the dressing. Serve immediately, while the potatoes are still warm.

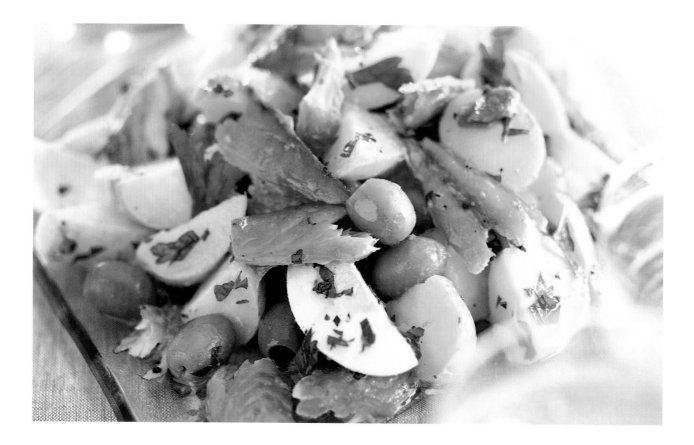

COD IN DILL SAUCE

Cod is very low in fat and a good source of protein, but it is quite a delicately flavoured fish. In this dish, the cod is served with a simple but tasty sauce.

1   Peel the cucumber and cut it in half lengthwise. Scoop out the seeds and discard. Chop the cucumber flesh into small chunks. Transfer to a bowl. Add the yogurt, mayonnaise and dill and mix together well. Season to taste. Cover and chill for at least 1 hour.

2   Place the fish in a sauté pan or deep, lidded frying pan and pour on the wine. Add enough water to ensure the fish is covered. Cover and place the pan over a medium-high heat. Bring to a boil then reduce the heat to low and simmer for 10 minutes until the fish flakes easily when tested with the tip of a knife.

3   Drain the fish, reserving 2–3 tablespoons of the cooking liquid. Stir this into the dill sauce to thin it a little; serve with the fish.

1 cucumber

100 ml plain yogurt

4 tablespoons mayonnaise

1 tablespoon chopped fresh dill

Salt and pepper, to taste

4 small cod fillets, about 150 g each

100 ml white wine

Serves 4

FLASH-FRIED PEPPERED TUNA

A simple but effective way to cook tuna that sears the fish and seals in the flavour of this low-fat dish.

1   Place the tuna in a shallow non-metallic dish. Mix the soy sauce and grated ginger together and pour over the fish. Cover and leave to marinate for at least 1 hour.

2   When ready to eat, dry the tuna steaks with paper towel and sprinkle with the pepper. Heat a cast iron skillet or heavy-based frying pan over high heat. Dry-fry the tuna for 2 minutes on each side.

3   Place a heap of shredded Chinese leaf and beansprouts on individual serving plates and place the tuna steaks on top. Leave for a minute or so, so that the fish relaxes and releases its juices; serve.

4 x 100–150 g fresh tuna steaks

4 tablespoons soy sauce

1 cm piece of ginger, peeled and grated

2 tablespoons freshly ground black pepper

200 g Chinese leaf, shredded

75 g fresh beansprouts

Serves 4

CHARRED SESAME CHICKEN

3 tablespoons olive oil

2 teaspoons ground cumin

½ teaspoon freshly ground black pepper

1 clove garlic, crushed

2 tablespoons finely chopped fresh parsley

Juice of ½ lime

Juice of ½ lemon

4 boneless chicken breasts

4 tablespoons sesame seeds

Serves 4

The chicken for this dish is marinated before cooking to give this low-fat meat added flavour. Serve with a tomato and basil salad for a simple lunch with a Mediterranean touch.

1 Mix the oil, cumin, black pepper, garlic, parsley and lemon and lime juice in a large non-metallic dish. Turn the chicken in the marinade and leave, skin-side down and covered, for at least 1 hour.

2 Place a cast iron skillet or griddle pan over a high heat. When the pan is almost smoking reduce the heat to medium and place the chicken in it. Cook for 7 minutes. Turn the chicken and cook for 7 minutes more, until cooked through.

3 When the chicken is cooked, sprinkle on the sesame seeds and leave in the pan for 30 seconds to release their flavour. Remove the chicken and sesame seeds from the pan and leave to rest for a few minutes before serving.

ORANGEY CHICKEN

Salt and pepper, to taste

4 skinless, boneless chicken breasts

Juice and zest of 2 oranges

4 tablespoons runny honey

½ teaspoon cayenne pepper

Serves 4

So simple to make, this is an ideal low-fat, light dish. Serve it with a leafy green vegetable or a few salad leaves for a perfect healthy lunch.

1 Season the chicken with salt and pepper and place in a large, shallow non-metallic baking dish. Mix together the orange juice, zest, honey and cayenne in a small bowl. Pour over the chicken. Turn the meat in the marinade to ensure it is well coated. Cover and leave to marinate for at least 1 hour.

2 Preheat the oven to 200°C, gas mark 6. Transfer the baking dish to the oven and bake for 45 minutes until the chicken is completely cooked through.

BARBECUED ORANGEY CHICKEN
Marinating is an ideal way to add flavour to chicken before cooking on a barbecue – the quick cooking time means there's little chance to introduce new flavours while the meat is being cooked. The marinade used in this dish gives the chicken a sweet orangey taste that will survive the intense heat of the barbecue. Cut the chicken into 3–4 cm cubes before marinating and then thread on to skewers to barbecue.

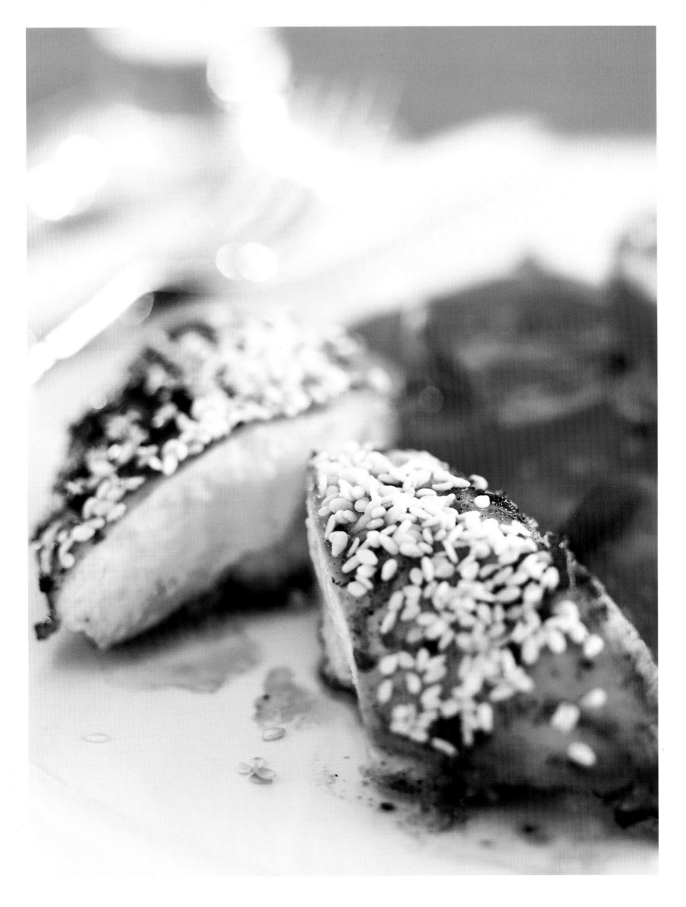

TURKEY STIR FRY

I large head of broccoli

4 spring onions

450 g skinless, boneless turkey breast, cut into strips

2 tablespoons rapeseed or sunflower oil

I large onion, finely sliced

I red pepper, finely sliced

I yellow or orange pepper, finely sliced

I courgette, sliced

2 cloves garlic, crushed

I tablespoon sherry

I teaspoon sesame oil

2 tablespoons soy sauce

50 g slivered or sliced almonds

Serves 4

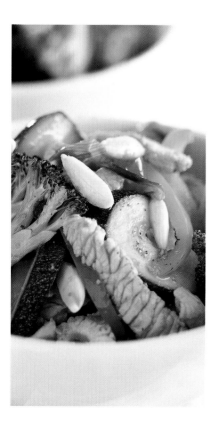

A tasty stir-fry packed with vegetables, the deep colours of the peppers and courgettes provide cancer-fighting substances. Serve it simply on a bed of plain boiled rice or with noodles.

1 Cut the broccoli into small florets and slice the spring onions into 1 cm long pieces. Place a non-stick wok or large non-stick frying pan over a high heat and dry fry the turkey in batches until browned; set aside.

2 Heat the rapeseed or sunflower oil in the same pan over medium heat and stir-fry the onion and peppers for 5 minutes. Add the broccoli and stir-fry for a further 5 minutes. Add the courgette and garlic and stir-fry for 3 minutes more.

3 Return the turkey to the pan and stir-fry over a medium-low heat for 5 minutes. Stir in the sherry, sesame oil and soy sauce and cook for a further 5 minutes, until the turkey is cooked through.

4 Stir in the spring onions. Transfer to individual dishes and scatter with the almonds to serve.

SPECIAL FRIED RICE

To make this recipe go further, serve it with a hearty rice accompaniment. Fried rice is made with cooked rice so you can use leftovers or pre-cook some, in which case you should prepare the rice the day before. Cook 50 g long-grain rice per person, drain and spread out on a baking tray to dry out. When you are ready to make the dish, peel and finely chop a 1 cm piece fresh ginger, finely chop 1 garlic clove and 4 spring onions, and finely slice 100 g mushrooms. Defrost 3 tablespoons frozen peas. Heat 2 tablespoons rapeseed or sunflower oil in a wok over medium heat and fry the ginger and garlic for about 30 seconds before adding the spring onions and mushrooms. Stir-fry for 3–5 minutes until the vegetables have softened. Add the rice and peas and cook for a few minutes more, stirring all the time, until all the rice is piping hot. Stir in 1 teaspoon sesame oil and 1–2 tablespoons soy sauce, to taste. Serve at once.

MARINATED SKEWERED TURKEY

This is a wonderfully light meat dish; the marinade helps keep the low-fat turkey moist and the honey adds just the right note of sweetness. Serve in pitta breads with a little shredded iceberg lettuce.

1 Cut the turkey into 4 cm cubes. Mix the marinade ingredients together in a large non-metallic bowl. Add the turkey and stir to coat all the pieces. Cover and leave in the fridge for at least 1 hour.

2 If using wooden skewers, soak them in water for 15 minutes to help prevent burning. Heat the grill to high.

3 Thread the turkey on to skewers. Place a little piece of foil on the tips of the skewers as these can burn, even if soaked. Grill for 7–10 minutes, turning regularly, until the turkey is cooked through and browned at the edges.

4 Put the pitta breads on the grill with the turkey while it is cooking and grill them lightly until they begin to puff up. Remove from the grill and leave to cool slightly before slitting open. Fill each one with shredded lettuce. Remove the turkey from the skewers and add to the pittas; serve.

750 g skinless, boneless turkey thigh meat

4 pitta breads

A few iceberg lettuce leaves, shredded, to serve

FOR THE MARINADE

2 cloves garlic, crushed

3 tablespoons clear honey

4 tablespoons tomato ketchup

4 tablespoons Worcestershire sauce

2 teaspoons mustard

2 teaspoons soy sauce

Serves 4

PORK ESCALOPES WITH HONEY & PECANS

A quick cooking method for a low-fat meat – this simple dish works well served with plain noodles and lightly stir-fried broccoli and spring onions.

1 Mix together the flour, salt and pepper in a shallow dish or plate. Dip the escalopes into the mixture until well coated. Heat the oil in a large frying pan over medium-high heat. Add the escalopes and fry for 5 minutes on each side until browned and cooked through. Set aside and keep warm.

2 Pour off any oil that remains in the frying pan. Add the honey to the pan and warm gently over low heat. Add the pecans and stir well, cook for a few more seconds then pour over the escalopes and serve at once.

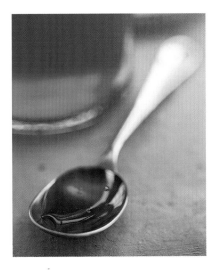

3 heaped tablespoons plain flour

Pinch of salt

1 teaspoon freshly ground black pepper

4 pork escalopes

2 tablespoons rapeseed or sunflower oil

4 tablespoons runny honey

100 g pecan halves

LAMB & HALLOUMI KEBABS

1 onion, finely chopped

Juice of 1 lemon

Freshly ground black pepper, to taste

800 g lamb fillet, cut into 3 cm cubes

3 courgettes

1 red pepper

1 yellow pepper

450 g halloumi cheese, cut into 3 cm cubes

Olive oil, for greasing

1 tablespoon finely chopped fresh mint

Serves 4

High in zinc and calcium, this dish is an aromatic Greek favourite that will keep the immune system and bones strong. Use good quality lean lamb that won't require long cooking.

1 Mix the onion with the lemon juice in a large non-metallic bowl and season with a little black pepper. Stir in the lamb, cover and leave to marinate for about 1 hour.

2 Preheat the oven to 230°C, gas mark 8. If using wooden skewers, soak them in water for 15 minutes to help prevent burning. Deseed the peppers and cut into 3 cm chunks and the courgettes into 5 mm thick slices.

3 Thread four skewers alternately with lamb, cheese, courgettes and peppers. Each skewer should take about three pieces of each. Place a little piece of foil on the tips of the skewers as these can burn.

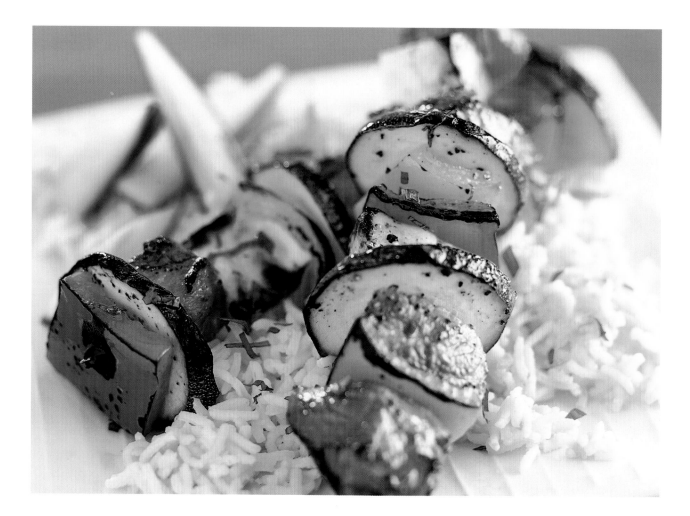

4   Line a shallow baking tray with foil and brush with a small amount of olive oil. Lay the kebabs on the tray and then brush them with a little oil, especially the cheese and vegetables. Bake on the top shelf for 15 minutes.

5   Meanwhile, heat the grill to its highest setting. When it is very hot, turn it down to medium heat. Finish off the kebabs under the grill for about 3 minutes to give them a charred appearance. Serve, sprinkled with the chopped mint.

LEMON GRASS BEEF WITH PAK CHOI

Leafy green vegetables and beef combine to create an iron-rich meal that's flavoured with a Thai-inspired marinade. Serve with plain boiled brown rice.

600 g sirloin or fillet of beef, trimmed of fat
1 lemon grass stalk
4 tablespoons fish sauce
2 tablespoons soy sauce
3 tablespoons lime juice
1 clove garlic, crushed
3 tablespoons flax oil
Freshly ground black pepper, to taste
2 small heads pak choi
1 red onion, thinly sliced
2 tablespoons rapeseed or peanut oil
Serves 4

1   Place the beef in the freezer for 30 minutes before you begin – it makes cutting the beef into fine slices much easier. Finely chop the lemon grass and mix with the fish sauce, soy sauce, 2 tablespoons lime juice and the garlic in a shallow non-metallic dish.

2   Cut the beef into very thin slices across the grain and add to the lemon grass marinade; mix well. Cover and leave to stand for at least 30 minutes.

3   To make the dressing, whisk the flax oil with the remaining lime juice and season with pepper. Separate the pak choi into leaves and and mix with the red onions in a large bowl. Pour on three quarters of the dressing and toss until the leaves and onions are well coated.

4   Heat the rapeseed or peanut oil in a large frying pan or wok over medium-high heat and stir fry the beef, working in batches if necessary, until it is done the way you prefer. (It will take about 1 minute for medium rare.)

5   Stir the cooked beef in with the dressed pak choi and onions. Drizzle with the remaining dressing and serve immediately.

PAK CHOI & PORK

This dish works well with pork – just use the same amount of tenderloin. You won't need to pop the pork in the freezer; it will be easier to slice than the beef. Cut across the meat widthways to get thin slices. Leave in the marinade for at least 30 minutes. Stir-fry for 3–5 minutes until the meat is cooked through. Serve as above.

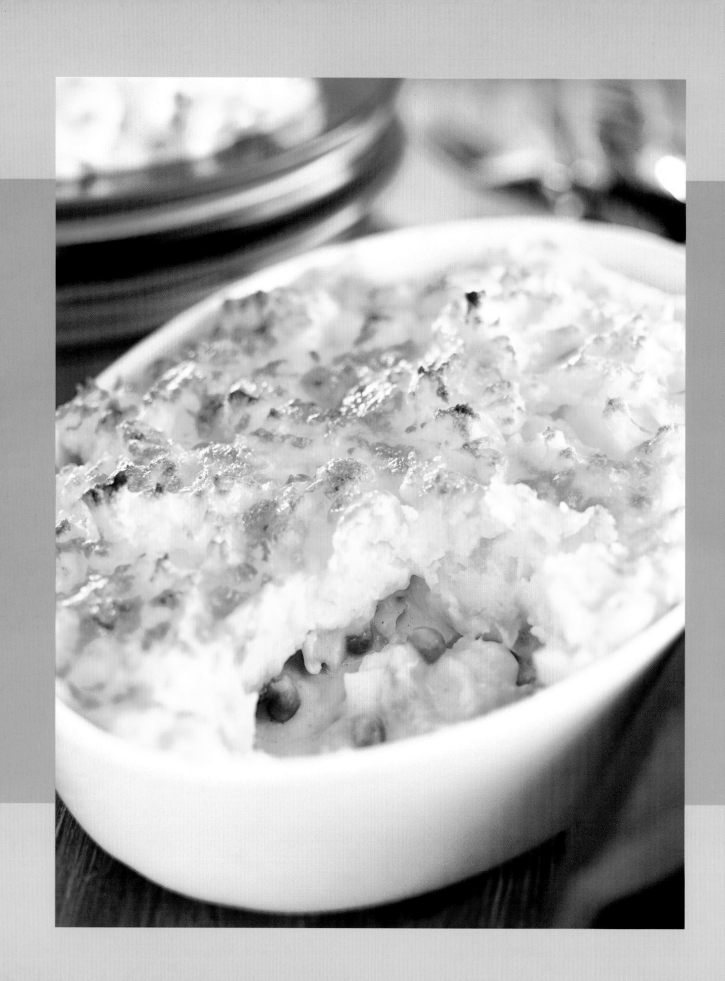

4 Main Courses

This chapter gives you a wide range of different dishes to choose from – whether you're looking for the main meal of the day or want something for a special occasion. There's a choice of vegetarian, fish and meat dishes – all packed with healthy ingredients.

RICOTTA & MUSHROOM CANNELLONI

Cheese, mushrooms and pasta combine to create a firm family favourite with the added benefit of being high in calcium.

2 tablespoons olive oil, plus extra for greasing

250 g large mushrooms, such as shitake, flat cap or portobello

2 x 250 g tubs of ricotta cheese

1 egg, beaten

75 g Parmesan cheese, grated

Salt and pepper, to taste

250 g lasagne

400 g can or jar of tomato pasta sauce

125 g mozzarella cheese, thinly sliced

Serves 4

1   Preheat the oven to 180°C, gas mark 5. Brush a large, shallow ovenproof dish with the extra oil.

2   Slice the mushrooms thickly. Heat the remaining oil in a large frying pan over a medium heat and fry the mushrooms for about 10 minutes, until they reduce in size and any moisture has evaporated.

3   Place the ricotta, egg and mushrooms in a large mixing bowl. Set aside 2 tablespoons of Parmesan, then add the rest to the bowl. Season to taste and mix together well. Set aside.

4   Fill a large pan with salted water and bring to a boil. Add sheets of lasagne a few at a time, to make sure they don't stick together. Boil the pasta for no more than 5 minutes – the sheets should be flexible but not properly cooked. Drain and rinse in cold water, making sure all the sheets are separate.

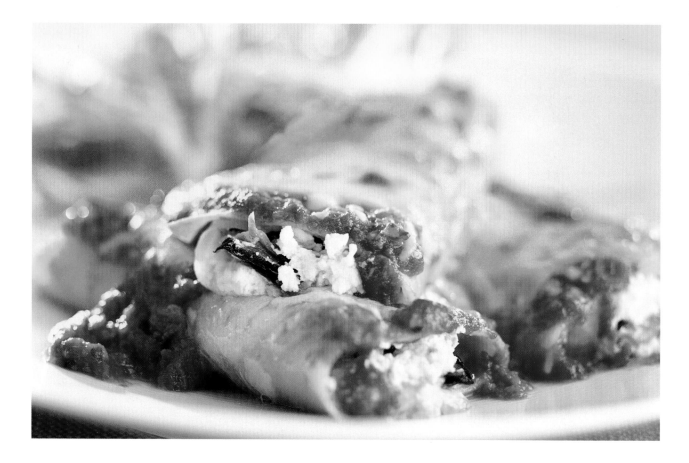

5 Lay out a sheet of lasagne and spoon 2 tablespoons of the ricotta mixture along one short edge. Roll it up and place in the greased ovenproof dish. Repeat with the remaining pasta sheets and ricotta mixture. There should be one layer only in your dish.

6 Pour the tomato sauce on top. Arrange the mozzarella on top of the tomato sauce. Sprinkle with the reserved Parmesan. Cover with foil and bake for 20 minutes. Remove the foil and bake for a further 20 minutes until the sauce is bubbling and golden.

LENTILS & RED PEPPER PASTA

Roasted red peppers and shitake mushrooms give this simple pasta dish a real depth of flavour. The recipe uses farfalle – bow-shaped pasta – but you could substitute any other flat pasta shape.

1 Preheat the oven to 200°C, gas mark 6. Cut the peppers in half and remove the seeds, pith and stalk. Lightly grease a baking tray with the extra oil. Lay the peppers on a baking tray and bake for 35 minutes. Using tongs, transfer the peppers to a polythene bag; seal and set aside.

2 Rinse and drain the lentils. Put them in a large saucepan with 1.2 litres water and place over medium-high heat; bring to a boil. Reduce the heat to low and simmer, uncovered, for about 25 minutes until tender but not soft.

3 Heat the oil in a large frying pan or sauté pan over medium heat and fry the onion for 3–4 minutes. Add the mushrooms and garlic and cook for a further 5–7 minutes until the mushrooms release their juices. Add the cooked lentils and warm through.

4 Remove the peppers from the bag and remove their skins; you should be able to rub them off quite easily. Roughly chop the flesh and stir in with the lentil mixture.

5 Meanwhile, place a large saucepan of salted water over medium-high heat and bring to the boil. Add the pasta and cook for 10–15 minutes. Drain and add to the pan with the lentil and pepper mixture. Stir well, over low heat, until everything is warmed through. Stir in the parsley and cheese and season with pepper to taste; serve at once.

2 red peppers

2 tablespoons olive oil, plus extra for greasing

200 g brown or green lentils

1 onion, finely chopped

125 g shitake mushrooms, roughly chopped

1 clove garlic, crushed

500 g farfalle

3 tablespoons finely chopped fresh parsley

3 tablespoons freshly grated Parmesan cheese

Freshly ground black pepper, to taste

Serves 4

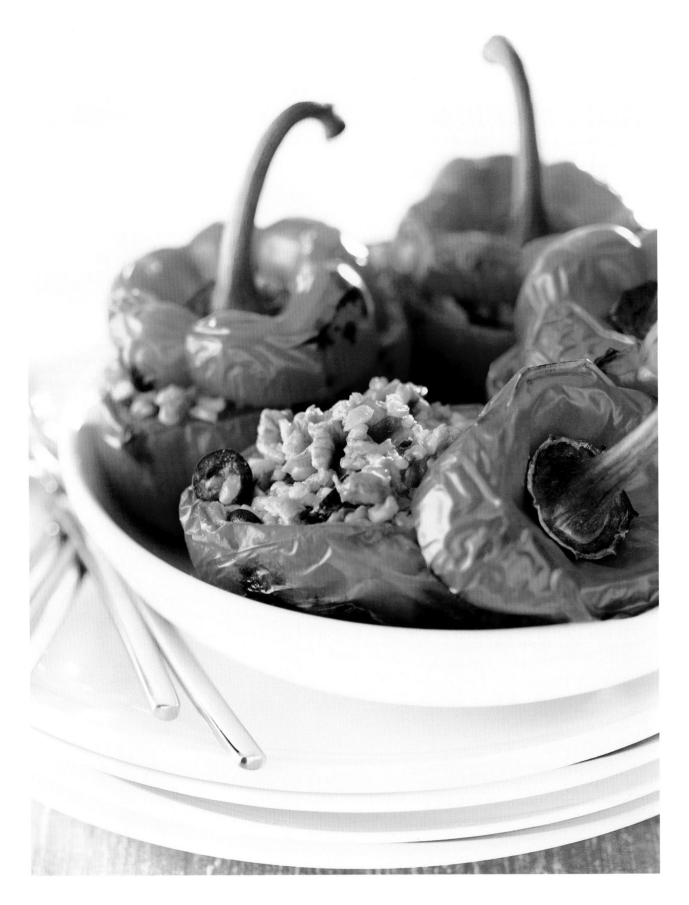

Risotto-stuffed Red Peppers with Walnuts & Olives

The goodness of brown rice and lots of tasty ingredients make a marvellous filling for red peppers. Filling and nutritious, these peppers need only a few salad leaves as an accompaniment.

1 Heat the grill to the highest setting. Carefully cut the tops off the peppers and reserve to use as lids. Remove the seeds and white membranes from inside the peppers and discard.

2 Grill the peppers and lids, turning them as necessary, until they are slightly softened and the skin is nicely charred all over. Set aside.

3 Pour the stock into a saucepan and heat over medium until hot. Turn the heat to low and keep the stock hot.

4 Preheat the oven to 180°C, gas mark 5. Heat the oil in a large saucepan over medium heat and sauté the onion for about 5 minutes until soft. Add the garlic and cook for 2–3 minutes more. Add the rice and sauté for a few seconds until the rice is well coated with the oil.

5 Use a ladle and spoon some of the hot stock into the saucepan with the rice. Continue to cook, stirring, until almost all the stock is absorbed. Continue adding the hot stock in the same way until only a couple of spoonfuls are left.

6 Add the chopped tomatoes and cook, stirring, until most of the tomato juice is absorbed. Test the rice – it should be tender but still firm to the bite. If it isn't done, add more of the hot stock. Stir in the olives, walnuts and cheese and season to taste.

7 Take a deep baking dish in which the peppers fit tightly when standing upright and grease with the extra oil. Fill the peppers with the rice mixture and place the reserved lids on top. Bake for 40 minutes then leave to cool slightly before serving.

4 large red peppers

1.25 litres vegetable stock

2 tablespoons olive oil

1 onion, finely chopped

2 cloves garlic, crushed

200 g Italian brown rice

225 g can chopped tomatoes

50 g black olives, pitted and sliced

50 g walnuts, chopped

100 g any strong hard cheese, cubed

Salt and pepper, to taste

Serves 4

RISOTTO WITH MUSHROOMS, BROAD BEANS & SAGE

A delicious risotto with mushrooms and high-fibre broad beans. Fresh sage is used as a flavouring, a herb that may help reduce night sweats and hot flushes.

100 g shelled broad beans

50 g butter

175 g shitake mushrooms, cut into small chunks

1 litre vegetable stock

1 large onion, finely chopped

280 g risotto rice, such as arborio

2 tablespoons chopped fresh sage

Shavings of Parmesan cheese, to serve

Serves 4

1   Fill a saucepan with water and bring to the boil. Cook the broad beans for 7–10 minutes, depending on their size. Drain and cool. Remove the grey-green outer skins and set aside.

2   Melt 25 g butter in a large saucepan and add the mushrooms. Cook over medium heat for at least 7 minutes until the mushrooms release their moisture and then re-absorb it, turning a dark golden colour and crisping slightly. Remove and set aside.

3   Pour the stock into a small pan and place over low heat; keep hot.

4   In the same pan used for cooking the mushrooms, melt the remaining butter over medium heat and cook the onion for 5 minutes, until softened. Do not allow to brown.

5   Stir in the rice, ensuring all the grains are covered with the buttery mixture. Add a few spoonfuls of the hot stock and stir well. Reduce the heat to just above a simmer and cook the rice, stirring, until almost all the liquid has been absorbed.

6   Add a few more spoonfuls of stock and repeat the process until all the stock is used up, continuing to stir the rice regularly. The whole process should take about 20 minutes. The rice will be soft to the bite, and the risotto should have a thick sauce-like consistency.

7   Stir the mushrooms, broad beans and sage into the rice. Serve topped with a few Parmesan shavings.

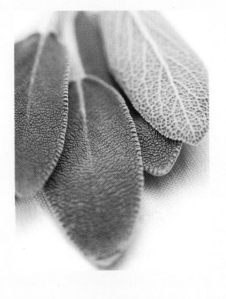

NUTTY BROWN RICE PILAU

Colours, textures and flavours make this a well-rounded nutritious favourite. Brown rice gives you more fibre than white and can make for a more filling meal.

1 Heat the grill to its highest setting. Line a baking tray with foil. Put the almonds and pine nuts on the prepared tray and toast under the grill for up to 2 minutes until just golden brown. Set aside.

2 Put the stock in a large saucepan and place over medium-high heat. Bring to a boil and add the rice. When the stock returns to the boil, reduce the heat to low. Cover and simmer for 30 minutes.

3 Meanwhile, heat the sesame oil in a large frying pan or wok over low heat and add the ginger. Fry gently for about 1 minute. Do not allow to burn. Add the spring onions, red pepper and mushrooms and stir-fry for 3–5 minutes. Stir in the soy sauce.

4 Stir the vegetables and the frozen peas into the rice. Cover again and cook on the lowest heat for another 10 minutes until the peas are defrosted and the rice is tender. Serve sprinkled with the almonds and pine nuts.

2 tablespoons slivered almonds

2 tablespoons pine nuts

600 ml vegetable stock

200 g brown rice

1 teaspoon sesame oil

2 cm piece fresh ginger, peeled and grated

3 spring onions, cut into 2 cm slices

1 red pepper, thinly sliced

200 g mushrooms, finely sliced

1 teaspoon soy sauce

4 tablespoons frozen peas

Serves 2–3

EGYPTIAN LENTIL PILAU

You can use white or brown rice in this dish, although brown is better, being higher in thiamine. Lentils are a good source of folic acid, copper and soluble fibre, as well as being a useful form of protein.

1 Rinse the lentils a couple of times. Put them in a large saucepan and cover with 600 ml water. Place over high heat and bring to a boil. Reduce the heat to low and simmer, uncovered, for 25 minutes until tender but not too soft; drain.

2 Meanwhile, pour 600 ml water into a large saucepan and place over high heat. Bring to a boil and add the rice and bouillon powder. Reduce the heat to medium-low, cover and simmer for 30 minutes until the rice grains are tender. Turn into a serving dish and mix with the cooked lentils. Leave to cool slightly.

3 Steam the diced courgette for a few minutes until just tender. Heat the oil in a small frying pan over medium-high heat and fry the onions for about 10 minutes until golden and crisp.

4 Stir the courgettes into the lentil and rice mixture and serve the pilau sprinkled with the crispy onions and parsley.

200 g brown lentils

200 g brown rice

1 tablespoon vegetable bouillon powder

1 yellow courgette, diced

2 tablespoons rapeseed or sunflower oil

4 large onions, finely sliced

3 tablespoons chopped fresh parsley

Serves 4

MUSHROOM STROGANOFF

2 tablespoons olive oil

3 onions, roughly chopped

1 clove garlic, crushed

2 teaspoons chopped fresh lemon thyme

Pinch of cayenne pepper

Pinch of ground cumin

500 g mixed mushrooms, such as chestnut, shitake and portobello, sliced

2 tablespoons tomato purée

400 ml vegetable stock

500 g fresh tagliatelle or linguine

100 g Greek yogurt, strained

1 tablespoon chopped fresh chives

Serves 4

A vegetarian pasta dish with a rich and filling sauce. Don't be tempted to use button mushrooms – they don't give the required colour, flavour or texture you need for this dish.

1　Heat the oil in a large frying pan over medium-low and fry the onions until they begin to turn golden in colour. Stir in the garlic, thyme, cayenne and cumin.

2　Add the mushrooms and cook over low heat for about 7 minutes until the mushrooms release their moisture and then re-absorb it, reducing in size by about two thirds.

3　Add the tomato purée and cook for a couple more minutes. Stir in the stock and bring to the boil. Reduce the heat to medium-low and cook for 10 minutes until the juices have evaporated by about a half.

4　Meanwhile, bring a large pan of salted water to the boil. Cook the pasta at a rolling boil for a few minutes until tender; drain. Stir the yogurt into the mushroom mixture and serve with the pasta, sprinkled with the chives.

COCONUT TOFU WITH PEANUT SPINACH

1 lime

2 teaspoons Japanese soy sauce

500 g tofu, drained and cut into 2 cm cubes

2 cloves garlic

2 cm piece of ginger

110 g shallots

3 tablespoons rapeseed or sunflower oil

1 piece of lemon grass, cut into 2 pieces

2 x 400 ml cans coconut milk

60 g fresh coriander, chopped

Tofu, or soya bean curd, is an ideal food for the menopause. It's a source of plant oestrogens and calcium and is low in fat. Serve it with plain boiled Thai fragrant rice to soak up the delicious sauce.

1　Take the lime and, using a potato peeler, cut off 3–4 long strips of zest; set aside. Squeeze out the lime juice and mix with the soy sauce in a non-metallic dish. Add the tofu, stir to coat well, and set aside for 5 minutes.

2　Meanwhile, peel and finely chop the garlic, ginger and shallots. Drain the tofu thoroughly, reserving the marinade, and pat dry with kitchen towel. Heat 2 tablespoons of oil in a wok or large frying pan over medium-high heat and fry the tofu, in batches, until golden brown all over. Remove from the pan and drain on a piece of kitchen towel.

3　Wipe out the wok or frying pan and add the remaining oil. Heat over medium-high heat and add the garlic, ginger and shallots. Stir-fry for 2–5 minutes until the shallots have become translucent. Add the reserved lime zest and pieces of lemon grass and stir fry for 30 seconds.

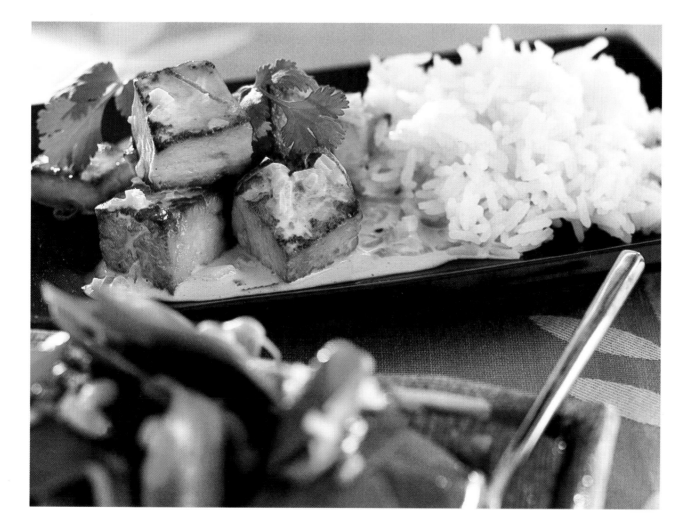

4 Pour in the reserved marinade and stir well. Pour in the coconut milk and bring to a rolling boil. Lower the heat and simmer, uncovered, for 10 minutes until the milk has thickened slightly. Stir in the tofu and continue to simmer for 15 minutes.

5 Meanwhile, roughly chop the peanuts. Place a heavy-based frying pan over medium-high heat. When the pan is hot, add the peanuts and dry-fry, stirring, for 5–10 minutes until the nuts are toasted; set aside to cool slightly. Roughly chop or tear the spinach into pieces and transfer to a serving bowl. Toss with the warm peanuts and the sesame oil.

6 When the tofu has finished cooking, remove the pieces of lime zest and lemon grass. Stir in the chopped coriander and serve immediately with the spinach.

FOR THE PEANUT SPINACH

60 g peanuts

115 g baby spinach leaves

2 teaspoons sesame oil

Serves 4

GRILLED FISH FLORENTINE

500 g fresh spinach

100 ml double cream

100 g Parmesan cheese, grated

Salt and pepper, to taste

4 small haddock fillets, about 150 g each

Serves 4

Here haddock is cooked with a creamy spinach sauce that keeps the fish moist and well flavoured. Although the sauce is fairly rich, the haddock is low in fat.

1　Wash the spinach very thoroughly and, with the water still clinging to the leaves, pack it into a large saucepan. Cook over high heat for 2–3 minutes until the leaves have wilted. Drain thoroughly and then chop it finely.

2　Mix the spinach, cream and cheese in a small saucepan and season to taste. Place over a low heat and cook, stirring regularly, until the cheese has completely melted and everything is well blended.

3　Heat the grill to high. Place the fish on a baking tray and grill, skin side up, for 2 minutes. Turn the fish over and grill for another 2–3 minutes, depending on the thickness of the fish. Cover the fillets with the spinach mixture and grill for a further 2–3 minutes until it is golden and bubbling and the fish is cooked through. Serve at once.

CRUSTY HALIBUT

115 g chopped walnuts

25 g fresh breadcrumbs

2 teaspoons paprika

1 teaspoon dried marjoram

½ teaspoon garlic salt

Freshly ground black pepper, to taste

1 large egg, beaten

4 halibut steaks

50 g butter

1 lemon, quartered, to serve

Serves 4

This tasty fish dish has a gently seasoned, nutty-crunch coating. Lovely with chips, it's served with lemon, cut into wedges to squeeze over the fish.

1　Grind the walnuts in a pestle and mortar or with a rolling pin on a chopping board – you want a coarse consistency, rougher than the breadcrumbs. Mix the breadcrumbs, paprika, marjoram and garlic salt with the walnuts and season with pepper. Pour onto a plate.

2　Place the beaten egg in a shallow bowl and dip the fish steaks first in the beaten egg and then into the nut-crumb mixture, pressing the mixture into the fish with your hands.

4　Melt the butter in a small frying pan over medium heat and fry the fish, skinless side down first, for 5 minutes. Then turn over and cook for another 5 minutes, skin side down.

5　Turn off the heat and leave the fish in the pan to rest for a couple of minutes. Serve with the lemon wedges.

SMOKED HADDOCK FISH PIE

*A real winter warmer, this potato-topped pie uses smoked haddock but
you could just as easily substitute the same amount of any firm-fleshed
fish, smoked or unsmoked.*

1   Cut one of the onions in half and cut the other into fine slices. Fill a small
pan with water and bring to the boil. Add the peas and cook for 1–2
minutes until defrosted. Drain and set aside.

2   Pour 300 ml milk into a sauté pan or large shallow saucepan and add the
fish and the two halves of onion. Cover the pan, place over a medium heat
and bring the milk to a boil. Reduce the heat and simmer for 20 minutes
until the fish has cooked through. Meanwhile, bring a large pan of water to
the boil and cook the potatoes for 15–20 minutes until just done; drain.

3   Heat the oven to 200°C, gas mark 6. Drain the fish, reserving the cooking
liquor (discard the onion). Flake the fish, removing the skin and any stray
bones, and transfer to a 2 litre pie dish or gratin dish. Mix in the peas.

4   Heat 25 g butter in a small frying pan over medium-low heat and fry the
sliced onion for 5–10 minutes until soft. Add the cumin and cook, stirring,
for 1 minute. Sprinkle on the flour and cook, still stirring, for another
minute. Gradually stir in the cooking liquor, a little at a time, until the
sauce is smooth and well blended. Bring to the boil, stirring constantly,
until the sauce has thickened. Reduce the heat to low and leave to simmer
for a couple of minutes. Season to taste and stir in with the fish.

5   Mash the potatoes with the remaining butter and milk and season to taste.
Spoon the mash on top of the fish mixture until it is completely covered.
Sprinkle with the grated cheese. Cook on the second shelf of the oven for
35–45 minutes until the topping is golden brown.

2 onions

100 g frozen peas

350 ml milk

1.5 kg smoked haddock fillet

1–1.2 kg floury potatoes, peeled and cut
into quarters

75g butter

½ teaspoon ground cumin

50 g plain flour

Salt and pepper, to taste

2 tablespoons grated double Gloucester

Serves 4

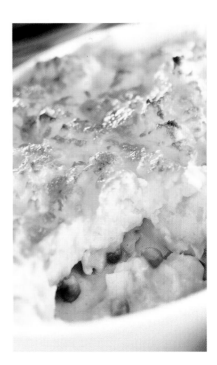

GRIDDLED SALMON WITH PARSLEY SAUCE

Eating more fish – especially fish high in Omega 3 oils – is one of the best things you can do to maintain a healthy heart, and salmon is a good source of this essential fatty acid.

½ slice wholemeal bread, crust removed

2 tablespoons lime juice

I clove garlic, crushed

2 tablespoons finely chopped or ground walnuts

4 tablespoons finely chopped fresh parsley

50 ml olive oil, plus extra for brushing

4 x 100 g salmon steaks or fillets

Freshly ground black pepper, to taste

Serves 4

1 Soak the bread in the lime juice for 10 minutes. Mash it up and mix in the garlic, walnuts and parsley. Gradually beat in the olive oil, adding only a little at a time. Leave to stand for 2 hours.

2 Brush both sides of the salmon with the extra oil and season with freshly ground black pepper. Heat a griddle pan until very hot and add the salmon. Cook on each side for 2–3 minutes then turn off the heat and leave the fish to rest for 2 minutes.

3 Meanwhile, transfer the sauce to a small saucepan and heat, stirring all the time, until nicely warm; do not allow to boil. Serve the salmon accompanied by the sauce.

CRUNCHY FILO SALMON

A perfect dish for entertaining, crispy filo pastry hides the meltingly tender flesh of the salmon – a real menopause super-food.

4 skinless salmon fillets

2 teaspoons chopped fresh sage

I teaspoon creamed horseradish sauce

I clove garlic, crushed

8 sheets filo pastry

2 teaspoons olive oil

Serves 4

1 Preheat the oven to 190°C, gas mark 5, and line a baking tray with foil. Place a frying pan over high heat and dry-fry the salmon for 2 minutes on each side until a little crust forms. Mix the sage, horseradish and garlic together and spread over the salmon fillets.

2 Lay a sheet of filo pastry on the work surface and brush with a little of the olive oil. Top with another sheet of filo pastry.

3 Lay one salmon fillet in the centre of the pastry. Lift the pastry over the salmon and scrunch up at the top, making sure the salmon is covered. Repeat with the remaining filo pastry and salmon fillets.

4 Transfer the filo parcels to the lined baking tray and place in the oven. Bake for 15 minutes until until the pastry is crisp and golden brown.

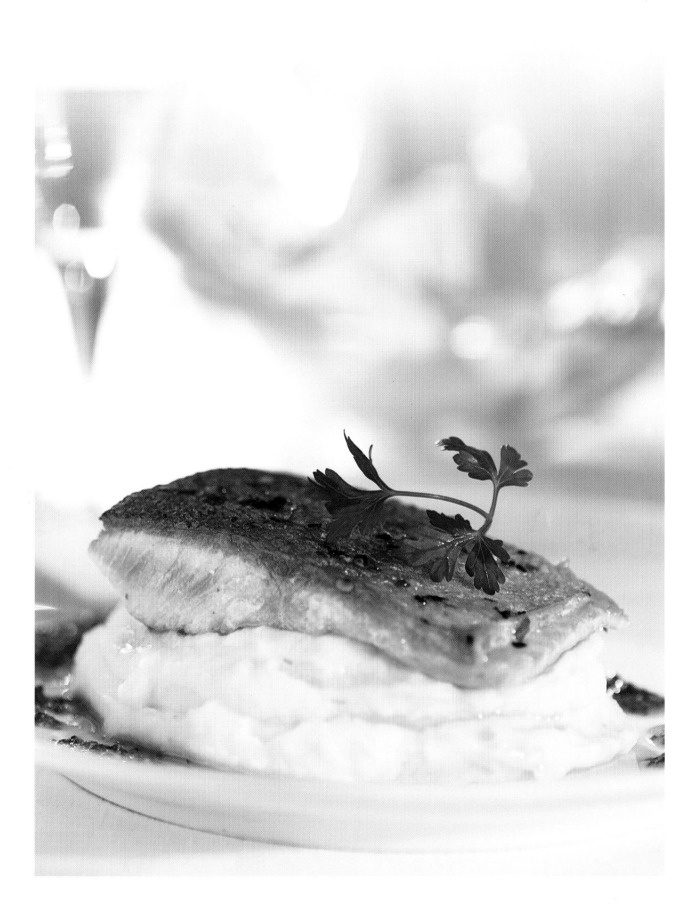

ROAST TROUT
WITH ALMONDS & HERBS

This classic recipe makes a wonderful dinner-party dish. The fish and nuts contain many essential fatty acids with a multitude of health benefits – they may help brain function and protect the heart.

4 trout, gutted and cleaned

2 tablespoons chopped fresh thyme

2 tablespoons chopped fresh parsley

2 tablespoons olive oil

2 limes

Salt and pepper, to taste

100 g flaked almonds

Serves 4

1 Preheat the oven to 230°C, gas mark 8. Wash the fish and dry them thoroughly, inside and out, with paper towel.

2 Mix the herbs, olive oil and juice of 1 lime together in a bowl and season to taste. Lay the fish on a baking tray and spoon the herb mixture inside the cavities, pouring any remainder over the skin.

3 Scatter the almonds on top of the fish. Transfer the baking tray to the second shelf of the oven and roast the fish for 25 minutes until cooked through. Serve with the remaining lime, cut into wedges.

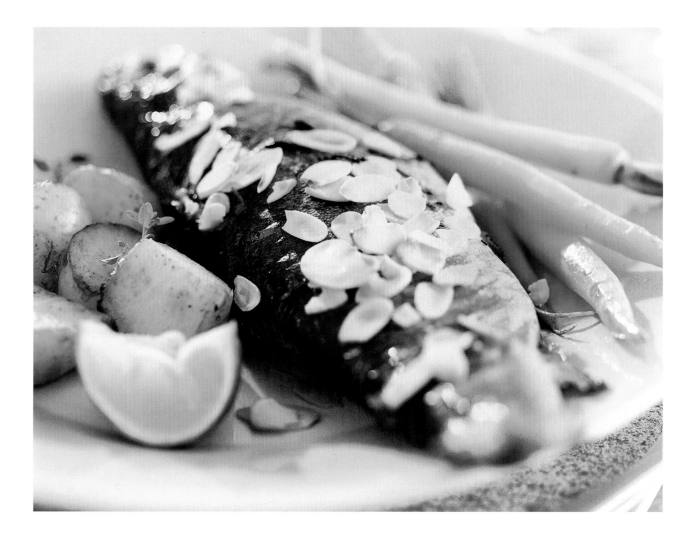

PRAWN PAELLA

Rice is mixed with prawns, tomatoes, green beans and olives to create a seafood version of this Spanish classic. Serve on its own or with a simple green salad.

1 Heat 2 tablespoons oil in a large saucepan and cook the onion for 3–4 minutes until it turns translucent. Add the rice, turn in the oil, then add the stock and bring to the boil. Reduce the heat to a simmer and cover the pan. Cook for 15–20 minutes until all the liquid is absorbed.

2 Remove the lid of the saucepan and stir in the tomatoes and olives. Continue to cook on a low heat until everything is piping hot.

3 Fill a medium-sized saucepan with water and bring to the boil. Trim the beans but leave them whole. Add to the boiling water and cook for 3–5 minutes until tender but still retaining some bite; drain and keep warm.

4 Put the remaining oil in a large frying pan and heat over medium. Add the garlic and chilli and fry for about 1 minute. Remove from the pan with a slotted spoon and add the prawns. Cook for 5–10 minutes until the prawns turn pink and are cooked through.

5 Pour the wine into the pan with the prawns. Let it bubble up for about a minute, then pour the contents of the pan into the rice; stir well. Stir in the herbs and serve at once with the cooked beans.

3 tablespoons olive oil

1 large onion, chopped

200 g long grain rice

500 ml vegetable stock

225 g can chopped tomatoes

50 g black olives, pitted and halved

300 g green beans

3 garlic cloves, sliced

½ fresh chilli, deseeded and cut into a few slices

16–20 large raw prawns, shelled

100 ml dry white wine

1 teaspoon chopped fresh coriander

1 teaspoon chopped fresh parsley

1 teaspoon chopped fresh basil

Serves 4

REGIONAL VARIATIONS

In Spain, there are as many different versions of paella as there are different regions, each version using popular local ingredients. So, in coastal areas you will find paellas made with fish and seafood, while inland you'll find chicken, rabbit and even snails. You can adapt this recipe in much the same way. Try adding some cooked chicken or some sliced Spanish sausage, such as chorizo.

SCALLOPS WITH WHITE WINE & PARSLEY

250 g fettuccine or linguine

1 tablespoon olive oil

Salt and pepper, to taste

8 scallops, with corals

1 clove garlic, crushed

½ fresh red chilli, deseeded and finely chopped (optional)

200 ml white wine

3 tablespoons chopped fresh parsley

1 tablespoon chopped fresh sage

Serves 2

This divine seafood dish is a delicious way to increase your zinc intake. Serve with a fine fresh pasta such as fettuccine or linguine. Omit the chilli if you have problems with hot flushes.

1   Fill a large saucepan with water and place over high heat. Bring to the boil and add the pasta. Cook, at a rolling boil, for 10–12 minutes until just tender; drain.

2   Meanwhile, heat the oil in a small frying pan over medium-high heat until very hot. Season the scallops and add to the pan with the garlic and chilli, if liked. Cook for 3–4 minutes, until the scallops are golden on one side.

3   Turn the scallops then pour in the wine, letting it bubble up. Stir and leave to cook for a further 2–3 minutes. Stir in the herbs and serve with the drained pasta.

SQUID WITH WHITE WINE & CORIANDER

For a cheaper alternative, why not try squid in this recipe? You'll need 2–3 squid per person. Buy gutted and cleaned squid, complete with tentacles. Cut the bodies into rings and trim the tentacles into manageable pieces. Heat the oil and cook the garlic and chilli as in step 2 and then add the squid. Cook for 3–5 minutes, stirring occasionally, until just cooked through but still soft. Pour in the wine and cook as in step 3. Add 3 tablespoons of chopped fresh coriander instead of the parsley and sage. And to accompany this dish, why not use noodles instead of pasta and serve with a few wedges of lime to squeeze over the squid?

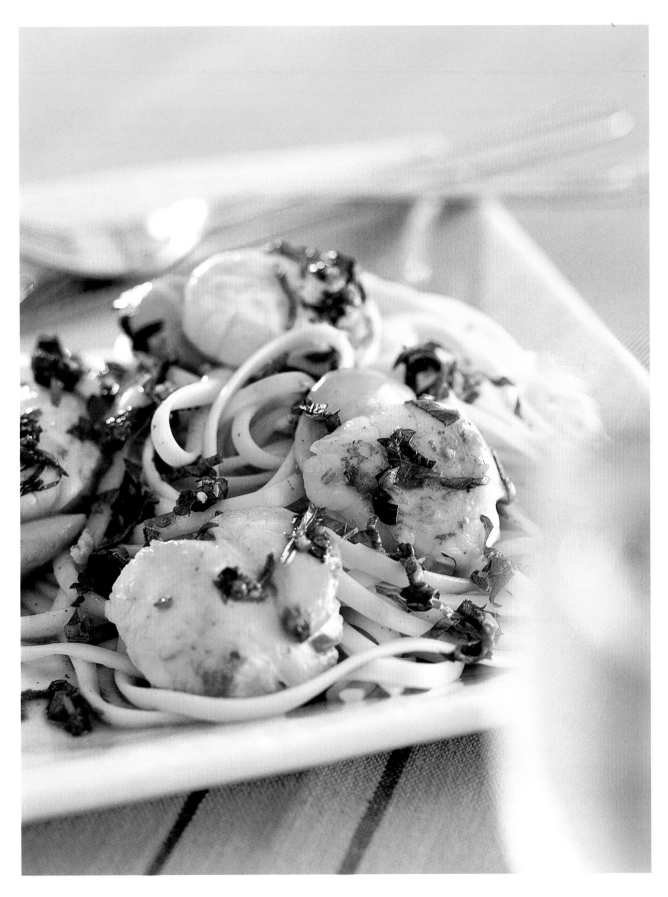

CIDER CHICKEN WITH TARRAGON

2 tablespoons olive oil

4 large onions, finely sliced

1.5–1.75 kg chicken, cut into 4 portions, or 4 large chicken quarters

2 tablespoons chopped fresh tarragon

400 ml cider

Serves 4

A delicious chicken dish, this is served with a rich, sweet, oniony gravy. Cook the chicken with its skin on for the best flavour – you can remove it to serve.

1 Heat the oil in a large sauté pan or deep, lidded frying pan and fry the onions, uncovered, over medium heat for at least 15 minutes, until golden in colour and sweet to the taste. Stir continuously and do not allow to brown too much.

2 Using a slotted spoon, remove the onions and keep warm, leaving the oil in the pan. Add the chicken to the pan and cook, skin side down, until golden. Then turn and cook for a couple more minutes.

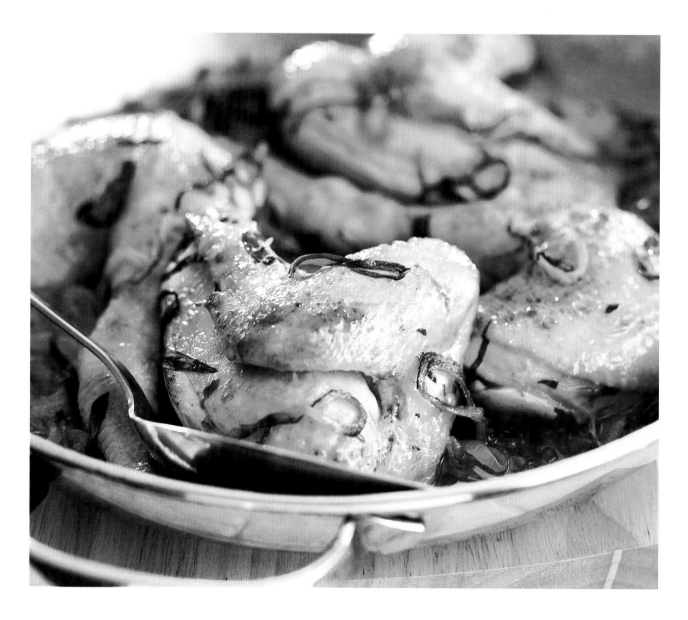

3   Stir in the onions and tarragon leaves, ensuring that there is at least a couple of spoonfuls of oil in the bottom of the pan. Cover and cook over medium-low heat for 20 minutes.

4   Remove the lid and add the cider. Turn up the heat until the liquid is boiling. Continue to boil for 5 minutes or until the liquid reduces by half – you will have a fine gravy rather than a thick sauce.

TURKEY PUFF PIE

A filling dish, perfect for winter's evenings, when you want something warm and satisfying to ward off the chills.

1   Preheat oven to 200°C, gas mark 6. Heat 2 tablespoons of oil in a large frying pan and cook the onion, carrot, celery and celery leaves for 7–10 minutes until soft. Turn the contents of the pan into a large baking dish.

2   Fill a small pan with water and bring to the boil. Add the peas and cook for 1–2 minutes until defrosted. Drain and stir in with the vegetables.

3   Put the turkey into a plastic bag with the flour and shake until well coated. Heat the remaining oil over a fairly high heat in the same frying pan as the vegetables and fry the turkey until browned on all sides, working in batches if necessary. Add to the cooked vegetables and mix together.

4   Mix the stock with the soy sauce and black pepper in a jug and pour into the hot frying pan. Stir well, scraping up any bits left on the bottom of the pan. Pour over the turkey and vegetables. Sprinkle with the thyme leaves.

5   Roll out the pastry, quite thinly, until slightly larger all round than the dish. Lay the pastry over the turkey and vegetables and brush with the beaten egg. Make a tiny cross in the middle of the pastry to allow air to escape.

6   Place the dish on a foil-lined baking tray to catch any drips and bake for 45 minutes until the pastry is puffed and golden. Leave to cool for a few minutes before serving.

3 tablespoons rapeseed or sunflower oil

1 onion, sliced

3 carrots, sliced diagonally

2 stalks celery, sliced diagonally

A few leaves from the celery, finely chopped

100 g frozen peas

450 g skinless, boneless turkey meat, cut into 3 cm cubes

2 tablespoons plain flour

300 ml vegetable stock

1 teaspoon soy sauce

1 tablespoon freshly ground black pepper

A few thyme leaves

375 g ready-made puff pastry

1 egg, beaten

Serves 4

ROAST DUCK
WITH PEACHES AND GINGER

4 duck breasts

100 ml orange juice

5 tablespoons soy sauce

4 tablespoons honey

4 cm piece of ginger, peeled and grated

1 teaspoon ground ginger

425 g can sliced peaches in syrup

100 g dried peaches or apricots, coarsely chopped

Serves 4

Duck breasts are the leanest cuts of duck and, as this recipe uses no extra fat, you can create a tasty dish that's lower in fat. The spicy sweetness of the ginger-flavoured marinade works well with the rich flesh of the duck.

1 Place the duck in a shallow non-metallic dish. Mix the orange juice, soy sauce, honey, grated ginger, ground ginger and half the syrup from the canned peaches together and pour over the duck. Sprinkle with the dried peaches. Cover and leave to marinate for at least 1 hour.

2 Preheat oven to 220°C, gas mark 7. Line a roasting tin with foil. Heat a cast-iron skillet or heavy-based frying pan until it is very hot. Drain the duck, retaining the marinade, and place it skin-side down in the hot pan. Dry-fry for about 3 minutes. Lower the heat and cook for another 10 minutes until the skin is dark and crispy. Drain off any fat.

3 Using a slotted spoon, remove the duck from the pan and transfer to the foil-lined roasting tin. Pour on the canned peaches and marinade. Roast for 30 minutes.

4 Allow to rest for 10 minutes before serving. Cut the duck breasts into fine slices to serve, removing the skin if wished, and accompanied by the cooking juices.

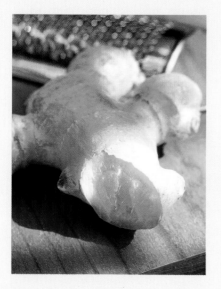

DUCK PANCAKES WITH CHUTNEY

Try this fresh way with an old take-away favourite and benefit from the iron and B vitamins in duck. Serve with simply cooked green beans or broccoli.

1 Place the duck breasts in a shallow non-metallic dish, skin side down. Pour over the soy sauce, cover and marinate for at least 1 hour.

2 To make the pancake batter, mix the milk with 125 ml water in a jug. Sift the flour and salt into a large bowl. Make a well in the flour and pour in the egg. Pour in half the milk and water mixture, a little at a time, beating the flour into the liquid with each addition. When all the flour is incorporated, whisk the batter until smooth. Set aside for a few minutes before adding the remaining milk and water mixture and the oil. Whisk the batter until it is slightly bubbly and has the consistency of single cream. Set aside for at least 30 minutes.

3 To cook the duck, preheat the oven to 220°C, gas mark 7. Place a cast-iron skillet or heavy-based frying pan over medium heat. When the pan is hot, dry fry the duck for at least 10 minutes on each side. When the skin is crispy, lift the duck out of the pan with a slotted spoon and place on a baking tray. Roast for 30 minutes or until cooked through. Remove the duck from the oven and leave to rest for 10 minutes.

4 Meanwhile, cook the pancakes. Lightly grease the base and sides of a frying pan with the extra oil and heat over medium-high. When the pan is hot, pour in enough batter to cover the base of the pan. Cook the pancake for about 2 minutes on one side until little bubbles begin to break through on the surface. Turn, and cook for about 30 seconds on the other side. Continue until all the batter is used up, re-greasing the pan as necessary. You should have enough batter for 8–12 pancakes. Keep the cooked pancakes warm.

5 Remove the skin from the duck and discard. Chop the flesh into bite-sized pieces. Transfer to a large bowl and mix with the chutney; season to taste. Take one pancake and place a couple of spoonfuls of the duck mixture, a handful of beansprouts and a few strips of cucumber in the centre; roll up. Continue until all the pancakes are filled with the duck, beansprouts and cucumber. Serve at once.

4 duck breasts

5 tablespoons soy sauce

5 tablespoons any fruit chutney

100–120 g fresh beansprouts

1 cucumber, deseeded and cut into very thin strips

Salt and pepper, to taste

FOR THE PANCAKES

300 ml milk

175 g flour

Pinch of salt

1 large egg, beaten

1 tablespoon rapeseed or sunflower oil, plus extra for greasing

Serves 4

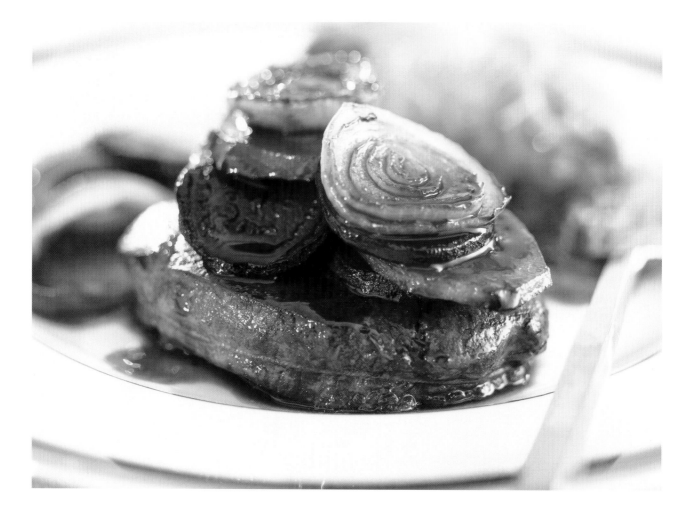

VENISON WITH ROOT VEGETABLES

2 venison fillets, about 200 g each

3 tablespoons olive oil

2 small raw beetroot, peeled and sliced

2 large potatoes, peeled and sliced

1 onion, peeled and sliced

100 ml red wine

70 g redcurrant or blackcurrant jelly

Salt and pepper, to taste

Serves 2

In common with the meat of most animals raised in the wild, venison is packed with healthy fats. It is also rich in iron. Serve with a bright green vegetable to complement the rich sauce.

1 Preheat the oven to 200°C, gas mark 6. Heat a cast-iron skillet or griddle pan until very hot and dry-fry the venison for 3 minutes on each side. Transfer to an ovenproof dish that is just large enough to hold the fillets.

2 Heat the olive oil over medium heat in the same skillet or griddle pan and add the beetroot, potatoes and onion. Cook for 2–3 minutes until slightly softened then stir in the red wine and redcurrant jelly.

3 Bring the sauce and vegetables to a boil and allow to bubble for about 3 minutes, then pour over the venison fillets. Cook, uncovered, in the oven for 30 minutes. Season to taste.

POT-ROAST PORK TENDERLOIN

A low-fat dish, this pork recipe uses sauerkraut, a type of pickled cabbage popular in eastern European cooking.

1 Place a cast-iron skillet or heavy-based frying pan over medium-high heat. When the pan is hot, dry-fry the pork until browned on all sides.

2 Transfer the meat to a large saucepan with a tightly fitting lid. Bring a kettle of water to the boil and pour over the meat until just covered. Stir in the bouillon powder or crumbled stock cube. Bring the liquid back to the boil, then reduce the heat to low and simmer, covered, for 25 minutes.

3 Stir in the cider vinegar, sugar and pepper. Season with a little salt and add the sauerkraut, potato and caraway seeds. Return to the boil then reduce the heat to low and simmer, covered, for another 30 minutes. Leave to rest for 10 minutes then carve the meat into slices. Serve accompanied by the sauerkraut and a little of the cooking liquor.

600 g pork tenderloin

1 tablespoon vegetable bouillon powder or 1 vegetable stock cube, crumbled

50 ml cider vinegar

1 tablespoon soft light brown sugar

½ teaspoon ground black pepper

Salt, to taste

400 g sauerkraut

1 potato, peeled and grated

½ teaspoon caraway seeds

Serves 4

PORK CHOPS WITH ARTICHOKES & OLIVES

Pork chops are served on a bed of ginger- and sesame-flavoured pak choi in this tasty suppertime treat. Trimming the chops makes for a lower fat dish.

1 Drain the artichokes then cut them in half and drain again on kitchen towel. Brush the chops with a little olive oil and season with the pepper. Heat a cast-iron skillet or heavy-based frying pan over high heat until it is smoking. Reduce the heat to medium-high and dry-fry the chops for 12–15 minutes on each side. Don't try turning the chops for at least 5 minutes or they will stick, although you can turn them regularly after that time. Trim the fat from the cooked chops and transfer to an ovenproof dish. Cover and keep warm in the bottom of the oven.

2 Pour the sherry into the hot pan, stirring to lift any crusty bits off the bottom of the pan. Bring the sherry to a boil and cook until reduced by one third. Stir in the artichokes, olives and cayenne and reduce the heat to medium. Cook for a couple of minutes to heat through; keep warm.

3 Wash the pak choi and place it, with any water that clings to its leaves, in a saucepan. Take the chops out of the oven and pour any juices that have been released from the meat into the saucepan. Return the chops to the oven. Stir the ginger and sesame seeds in with the pak choi and cook over high heat for 1–2 minutes until the leaves have wilted. Serve the chops on top of the pak choi and spoon on the artichokes, olives and sauce.

300 g canned artichokes

4 pork chops

Olive oil, for brushing

Freshly ground black pepper to taste

200 ml sherry

10-12 black olives, pitted

Pinch of cayenne pepper

2 heads pak choi

2 cm piece fresh ginger, peeled and grated

4 teaspoons sesame seeds

Serves 4

RÖSTI PORK

This is a delicious winter recipe, a variation on the old favourite, shepherd's pie. It's finished with potato rösti, rather than the traditional mashed potato.

2 tablespoons olive oil

1 onion, finely chopped

1 clove garlic, crushed

450 g minced pork

400 g can chopped tomatoes

1 tablespoon passata or sieved tomatoes

Pinch of sugar

2 tablespoons fresh thyme leaves

1 Preheat oven to 200°C, gas mark 6. Heat the oil in a large saucepan or sauté pan over medium heat and cook the onion and garlic for about 5 minutes until softened.

2 Add the pork and continue to cook, stirring regularly to break up the meat, for a further 5 minutes until the meat has browned completely. Spoon off any fat then add the tomatoes, passata, sugar and thyme leaves. Bring to a boil then reduce the heat and leave to simmer for 15 minutes until most of the liquid has evaporated.

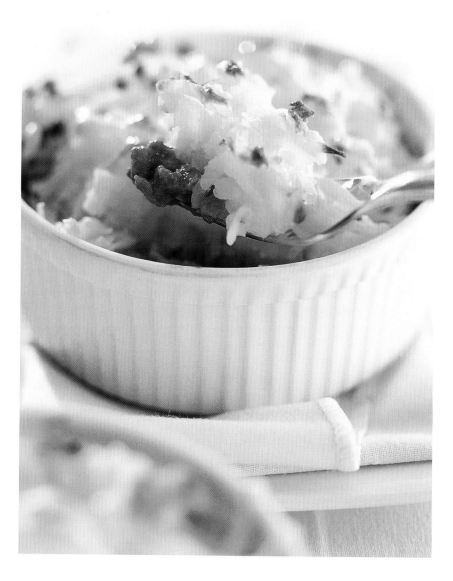

3 Meanwhile, bring a large saucepan of water to the boil and add the potatoes, still in their skins. Boil for 20 minutes until tender. Drain and, when cool enough to handle, peel off the skin and grate the potato into a bowl to make the rösti topping; season to taste.

4 Place the pork and tomato mixture in a 2-litre gratin dish or pie dish. Cover thickly with the rösti topping. Bake in the oven for about 30 minutes, until the rösti topping has turned golden brown. Sprinkle with the cheese, if liked, and place the dish under a hot grill for just a few seconds before serving to allow the cheese to bubble up.

FOR THE TOPPING

900 g floury potatoes

Salt and pepper, to taste

50 g Gruyère cheese, grated (optional)

Serves 4

LAMB TAGINE WITH APRICOTS

A delicious meaty dish that's a good source of iron, zinc and B vitamins. Even the dried apricots are a good source of iron.

1 Preheat the oven to 170°C, gas mark 3. Place a large cast-iron skillet or large heavy-based frying pan over medium-high heat. When the pan is hot, dry-fry the lamb in batches until browned all over. Transfer to an ovenproof casserole dish.

2 Heat the oil in the same pan over medium heat and add the onion. Cook for 2–5 minutes until the onion is translucent. Add the garlic, cinnamon, cumin and turmeric and cook for a further 5 minutes.

3 Add the lemon juice, stock, wine and dried apricots to the frying pan and season with the pepper to taste. Bring to a boil then pour the contents of the pan into the casserole with the lamb. Cover and cook 1½ hours until the meat is tender.

800 g lamb fillet, cut into 3 cm cubes

2 tablespoons olive oil

2 onions, roughly chopped

3 cloves garlic, crushed

4 teaspoons ground cinnamon

2 teaspoons ground cumin

1 teaspoon turmeric

Juice of 2 lemons

200 ml vegetable stock

500 ml red wine

350 g dried apricots, chopped

Freshly ground black pepper, to taste

Serves 4

LAMB KOFTAS

Rapeseed or sunflower oil, for greasing

700 g minced lamb

2 onions, finely chopped

2 tablespoons finely chopped fresh sage

1 teaspoon ground cumin

Salt and pepper, to taste

Serves 4

A particularly tasty way to eat lamb – baking the koftas allows the meat to release most of its fat and become a lower-fat dish. Serve with pittas, humous and a few slices of red onion.

1   If using wooden skewers, leave them to soak for at least 15 minutes to prevent them burning later.

2   Preheat the oven to 230°C, gas mark 8. Cover a baking tray with foil and grease the foil with oil.

3   Mix the lamb with the onion, sage and cumin in a large bowl; season to taste. Wetting your hands first, form the mixture into sausage shapes around the skewers. Cover the tips of wooden skewers with foil.

4   Lay the skewers on the greased foil. Bake on the top shelf of the oven for 20 minutes, draining off the fat regularly. Remove any foil from the skewers' tips and serve.

LAMB CASSOULET

800 g lamb fillet, cut into 3 cm cubes

2 tablespoons olive oil

1 onion, sliced

1 clove garlic, crushed

2 x 400 g cans chopped tomatoes

250 ml red wine

300 ml vegetable stock

2 teaspoons chopped fresh rosemary

1 tablespoon passata or sieved tomatoes

Freshly ground black pepper, to taste

2 x 450 g cans cannellini beans, rinsed and drained

Serves 4

Real comfort food, this cassoulet combines lamb with energy-boosting beans. Serve with a bright green vegetable like broccoli, curly kale or lightly steamed shredded Savoy cabbage.

1   Preheat the oven to 170°C, gas mark 3. Place a large frying pan over high heat and when the pan is hot, quickly dry-fry the lamb, in batches, until browned on all sides. Transfer to an ovenproof casserole.

2   Using the same frying pan, heat the oil over medium heat and gently cook the onion and garlic for about 5 minutes, without browning.

3   Add the tomatoes, wine, stock, rosemary and passata; season with pepper to taste. Stir well, scraping up any bits of lamb left in the pan. When the liquid begins to bubble, pour into the casserole dish.

4   Cover the casserole dish and cook in the oven for 1 hour. Add the beans and cook uncovered for another 20–30 minutes until the liquid has reduced by a third; serve.

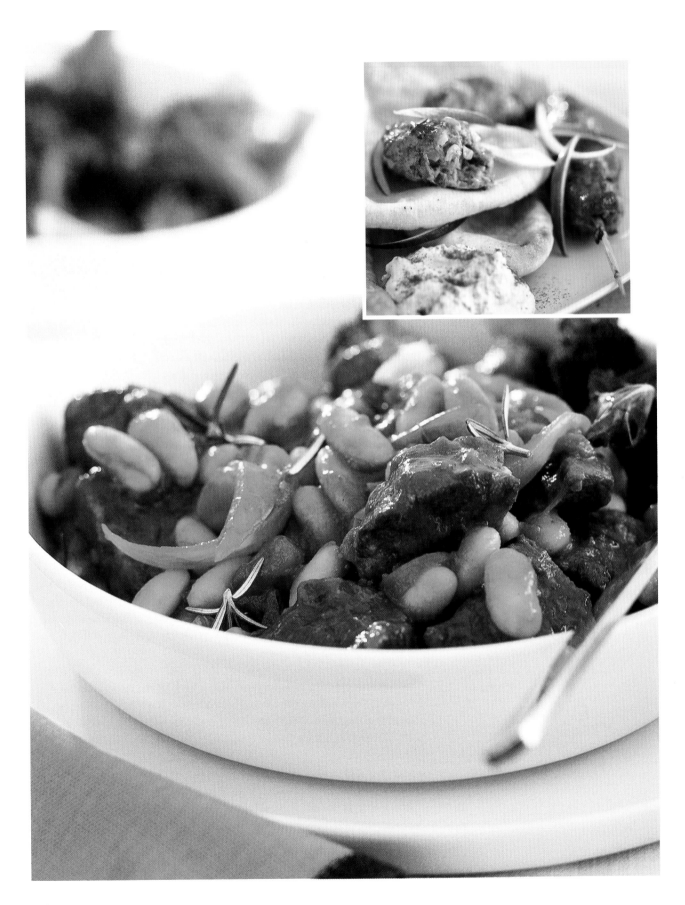

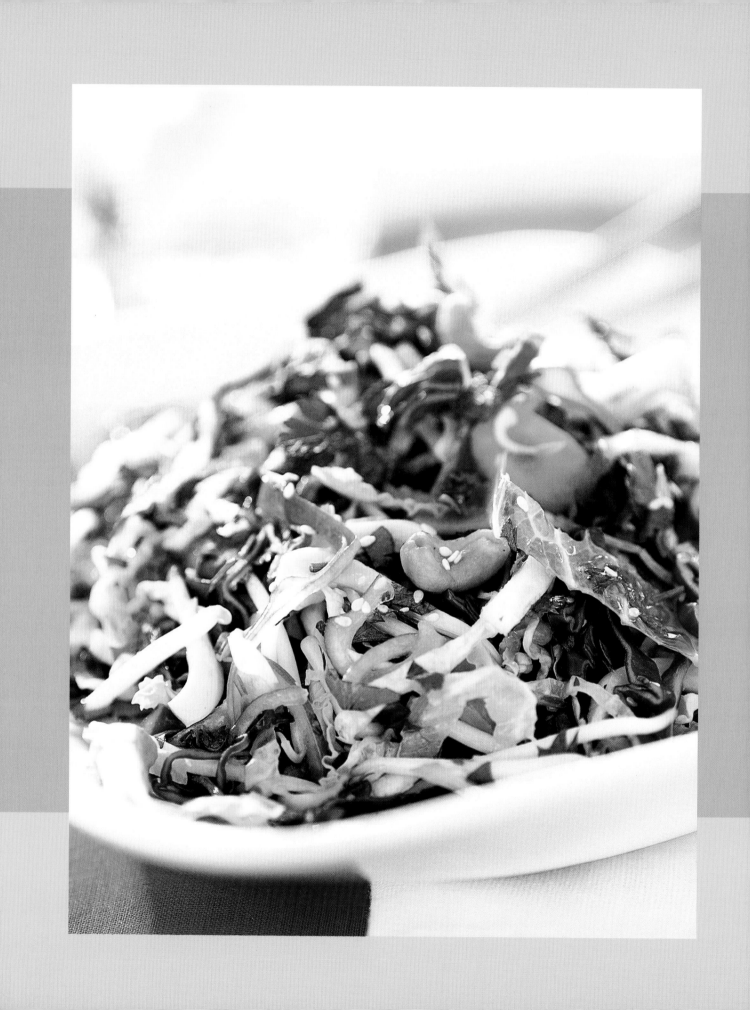

5 Side Orders

Make the most of your food's potential and serve meals that are as nutritious as possible. This chapter looks at ways to create delicious side dishes that are as healthy as they are tasty.

BRAISED CELERY WITH ALMONDS

50 g almonds, skinned

6 celery stalks (white if possible)

2 tablespoons olive oil

110 ml vegetable stock

Salt and pepper, to taste

Serves 4

Usually the preserve of salads, celery makes a delicious cooked accompaniment – especially when combined with the extra goodness of the almonds and olive oil.

1 Preheat the grill to its highest setting. Scatter the almonds on a baking tray and toast under the grill for just a few seconds until golden; set aside. Slice each celery stalk diagonally into 2 cm pieces.

2 Heat the oil in a medium-sized frying pan and add the celery. Sauté for a few minutes then add the vegetable stock and season to taste. Bring to a boil then turn the heat down to low, cover the pan and simmer for about 10 minutes. The celery should still retain some crispness.

3 Serve immediately sprinkled with the toasted almonds.

BRAISED FENNEL & ONION

1 fennel bulb

2 small onions

1 tablespoon olive oil

1 clove garlic, crushed

2 tablespoon soy sauce (optional)

Salt and pepper, to taste

½ red pepper, finely chopped, to garnish

Serves 4

Fennel has distinct flavour and gentle braising brings out the best in this under-rated vegetable. Cooked with onions it makes a great accompaniment to fish dishes.

1 Cut the fennel bulb in half and and cut out the core; discard. Then cut each half diagonally into thin slices. Peel and slice the onions into thin rings.

2 Fill a medium-sized saucepan with water and place over medium-high heat. Bring to the boil and add the fennel. Cook for 2–3 minutes; drain.

3 Pour the oil into a wok or large frying pan and place over medium heat. Add the onions and cook for 2–3 minutes, until they are translucent and turning slightly golden in colour. Add the fennel, garlic and soy sauce (if using) and cook for another 3–4 minutes. Season to taste. Cover the pan, reduce the heat to low and cook for another 2–3 minutes.

4 Serve at once, garnished with with the finely chopped red pepper.

ARMENIAN POTATOES

A potato dish with real flavour, this is the ideal accompaniment to plainly grilled or roast meats. Potatoes contain potassium, which can help reduce blood pressure.

1 Preheat the oven to 220°C, gas mark 7. Peel and cut the potatoes into 2 cm dice and rinse thoroughly in a colander. Mix the oil, tomato purée, paprika and garlic with 125 ml water in a measuring jug. Set aside some of the parsley to garnish, then stir the rest into the jug.

2 Turn the potatoes into a large roasting tin or baking tray. Pour the oil and tomato purée mixture over the potatoes and, using your hands, mix well until the potatoes are thoroughly coated. Season with salt and pepper.

3 Cover the tin or tray with a large sheet of foil, tucking it in well around the edges, and bake for 1 hour until the potatoes are soft. Cook, uncovered, for a further 15 minutes until the edges of the potatoes are crispy. Sprinkle with the reserved parsley to serve.

750 g potatoes

125 ml olive oil

3 tablespoons tomato purée

1 teaspoon paprika

4 cloves garlic, crushed or finely chopped

3 tablespoons finely chopped fresh parsley

Salt and freshly ground pepper, to taste

Serves 4

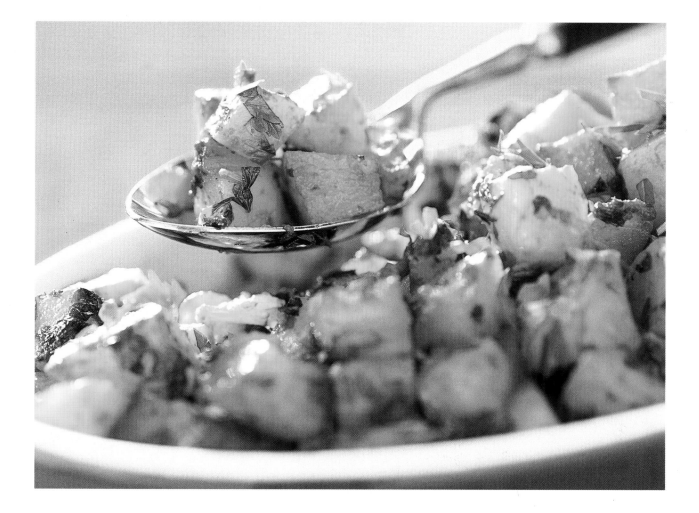

GREEN & WHITE SALAD

250 g runner or green beans

600 g canned cannellini beans

50 g pine nuts

FOR THE DRESSING

100 ml olive oil

2 teaspoons mild mustard

1 onion, grated

3 tablespoons chopped fresh parsley

3 tablespoons chopped fresh sage

Salt and freshly ground black pepper,
to taste

Serves 4–6

This fresh, tasty salad is packed with goodness – the beans are a delicious way to eat more fibre while the pine nuts are a good source of vitamin E.

1   Top and tail the beans, removing any stringy parts at the side if using runner beans, and slice. Bring a pan of salted water to the boil and add the beans. Bring back to the boil and cook for 3 minutes. Turn into a colander and rinse immediately under cold running water; drain and cool.

2   Drain the cannellini beans and rinse in a colander. Place in a serving bowl and mix in the cooled cooked runner or green beans.

3   Mix the dressing ingredients together in a jug and stir, with the pine nuts, into the vegetables. Serve at room temperature.

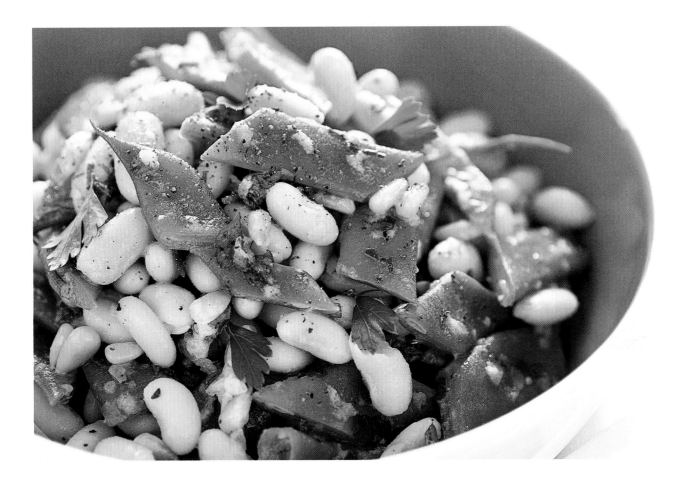

BUTTER BEANS IN CREAMY MUSTARD SAUCE

A luxurious and flavoursome side dish, made with butter beans – a great source of fibre – in a rich, creamy sauce.

1 Rinse and drain the beans in a colander, shaking off as much water as possible.

2 Heat the oil in a medium-sized saucepan over medium heat and fry the onion for a few minutes; do not allow to brown. Add the beans and wine and bring to a boil. Reduce the heat and simmer for about 15 minutes.

3 When the liquid has evaporated by half, add the cream and mustard. Bring back to the boil, then immediately reduce the heat to low and simmer for 2–3 minutes.

4 Stir in the cheese, season with black pepper and serve immediately.

400 g can butter beans

2 tablespoons rapeseed or sunflower oil

1 red onion, finely chopped

100 ml white wine

100 ml double cream

2 teaspoons mild mustard

50 g grated Cheddar

Freshly ground black pepper, to taste

Serves 2

LEMON SAGE PEAS

A herby way with peas that's low in salt and which turns a humble but ever-popular vegetable into an exceptional side dish.

1 Put the butter in a medium-sized saucepan and melt over gentle heat. Add the peas, herbs, lemon juice and 50 ml water. Turn up the heat and bring to the boil. Reduce the heat to low and cook, uncovered, for 5 minutes. Do not overcook as the peas will lose their bright colour.

2 Drain the peas, reserving the cooking liquor. Turn half the peas into a serving dish and keep warm. Transfer the remainder into a processor or blender and add the cooking liquor. Liquidise then pour over the peas in the serving dish, stir to mix.

3 Serve immediately, sprinkled with black pepper.

50 g butter

400 g frozen peas

1 tablespoon finely chopped fresh sage

1 tablespoon finely chopped fresh mint

2 tablespoons lemon juice

Freshly ground black pepper, to serve

Serves 4

CHICKPEA MASH

400 g can chickpeas

2 cloves garlic, crushed

50 ml olive oil

Salt and pepper, to taste

2 teaspoons snipped fresh chives

Serves 4

This flavoursome Mediterranean-style accompaniment makes a tasty alternative to mashed potato or rice. Chickpeas are a good, dairy-free source of calcium.

1 Rinse and drain the chickpeas in a colander, shaking off as much water as possible.

2 Put the chickpeas in a food processor with the garlic and blend. Then add half the oil and blend again. Season with salt and pepper to taste.

3 Empty the chickpea mash into a small saucepan and warm through gently for a few minutes – do not allow the mixture to boil. Stir in a little of the remaining oil while it is warming, until the mash has a silky texture. You may find that you do not need to add all the oil that's left.

4 Sprinkle with the snipped chives to serve.

CAULIFLOWER WITH PECANS

I small cauliflower

60 g pecan halves

2 tablespoons rapeseed or sunflower oil

3 spring onions, cut diagonally into 2 cm pieces

50 ml vegetable stock

I tablespoon soy sauce

I teaspoon sesame oil

Serves 4

Cauliflower is one of the crucifer vegetables – that contain cancer-fighting components and which are well worth including in any well-balanced diet.

1 Cut off the thick stems of the cauliflower and divide into florets. Heat a cast-iron skillet or heavy-based frying pan over medium heat. When the pan is hot, dry-fry the pecans for a minute or so until they give off an aroma. Set aside to cool.

2 Fill a medium-sized saucepan with water, place over high heat and bring to the boil. Add the cauliflower to the pan and cook for 3 minutes at a rapid boil. Drain thoroughly.

3 Heat the oil in a large frying pan or wok over medium heat and add the spring onions and cauliflower. Cook for a few minutes then stir in the cauliflower. Add the stock and soy sauce and bring to the boil. Reduce the heat to low, cover and cook for 2–3 minutes. Stir in the sesame oil and serve immediately sprinkled with the pecans.

BROCCOLI IN BLACK BEAN SAUCE

Quick cooking techniques allow you to get the best out of vegetables – and they give tastier results anyway. Broccoli is high in calcium for a vegetable, and another one of the cancer-busting crucifers.

1 Bring a pan of salted water to the boil and cook the broccoli for 2–3 minutes, making sure it retains its bright colour; drain.

2 Heat the oil in a large frying pan or wok and stir in the drained broccoli; stir fry for 1 minute over medium-high heat. Add the garlic, ginger, black bean sauce and sesame oil. Cook on a medium heat for 3 minutes allowing the sauce to bubble and cook through. Sprinkle with the sunflower seeds and serve immediately.

250 g broccoli florets
2 tablespoons rapeseed or sunflower oil
1 clove garlic, crushed
1 cm piece fresh ginger, peeled and grated
2 tablespoons black bean sauce
½ teaspoon sesame oil
2 teaspoons sunflower seeds
Serves 4

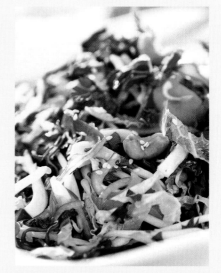

COLOURFUL CABBAGE SALAD

Eating a wide range of different coloured vegetables will increase the range of phyto-chemicals in your diet – substances that can help combat cancer and heart disease.

1 Peel the carrot and cut into very thin slices. Finely shred the cabbages. Combine the carrot, cabbages, beansprouts and onion in a large salad bowl.

2 Stir in the chopped herbs, nuts and sesame seeds. Drizzle on the sesame oil and toss the salad. Serve immediately.

COLOURFUL DRESSING

To make a light but tasty dressing for this salad, squeeze the juice of a lime into a jug and add 1 tablespoon rapeseed or sunflower oil, 1 tablespoon sesame oil, 2 tablespoons soy sauce, 1 crushed clove of garlic and a tablespoon of caster sugar. Whisk together well, ensuring the sugar is dissolved. Pour over the salad instead of the sesame oil in step 2 and toss everything together well.

1 large carrot
125 g each of red, white and green cabbage
125 g beansprouts
1 red onion, thinly sliced
2 tablespoons chopped fresh parsley
2 tablespoons chopped fresh coriander
50 g cashews or peanuts
1 teaspoon sesame seeds
1 tablespoon sesame oil
Serves 6–8

SHREDDED SESAME CABBAGE

I red pepper

I yellow pepper

2 tablespoons rapeseed or sunflower oil

I onion, sliced

2 cloves garlic, crushed

2 cm piece fresh ginger, peeled and grated

I green or Savoy cabbage, shredded

I teaspoon sesame oil

Serves 4

This aromatic and colourful accompaniment is an ideal healthy side dish and the quick cooking method is a good way to preserve much of the nutrients in the vegetables.

1 Cut the peppers in half and remove the seeds and pith; cut into slices. Heat the oil in a large frying pan or wok. Add the onion and stir fry for a couple of minutes.

2 Add the red and yellow pepper slices and stir fry for 2–3 minutes until slightly softened. Add the garlic, ginger and cabbage and stir fry for about 5 minutes more. Stir in the sesame oil and serve immediately.

ROAST CARROT & BEETROOT

4 large carrots

2 small raw beetroots

3 tablespoons olive oil

Salt, to taste

I teaspoon freshly ground black pepper

I tablespoon finely chopped fresh sage

I tablespoon finely chopped fresh basil

I tablespoon finely chopped fresh thyme

I tablespoon finely chopped fresh parsley

Serves 4

A well-flavoured side dish that's spectacularly coloured – with the reddy purple of the beetroot and orange of the carrots – and high in betacarotene.

1 Preheat the oven to 200°C, gas mark 6. Peel the carrots and slice them diagonally. Peel the beetroot and cut into 3 cm chunks.

2 Spread out the carrot and beetroot in a shallow baking or roasting tin and drizzle the oil over them. Sprinkle with a little salt and the pepper.

3 Roast for 30 minutes until the vegetables are tender, turning them in the oil half way through the cooking time. Mix in the fresh herbs and serve, accompanied by the cooking juices.

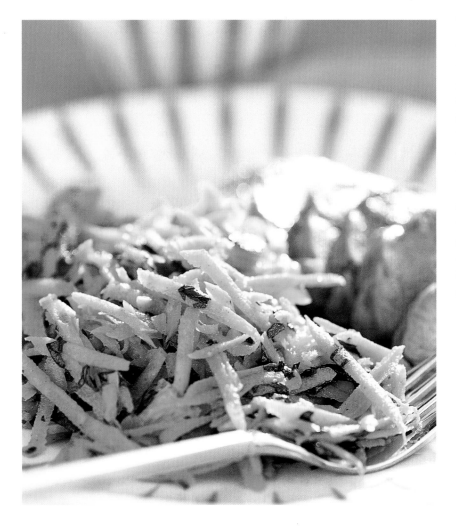

SANDWICH FILLING
You can use this recipe to make a tasty filling for sandwiches and other snacks. Mix the grated carrot with the orange flesh but omit the juices. Stir in the spices and add just 1 tablespoon of olive oil – leave out the lemon juice all together. Mix in the herbs just before serving.

Use as a filling for pitta bread; spread the inside of a pitta pocket with humous and fill with the carrot salad. Alternatively, team with a crumbly blue cheese and thick crusty bread for a cheese sandwich with an extra crunchy texture.

CITRUS CARROT SALAD

So simple and yet so tasty, this side dish is a great way to eat carrots – high in vitamin A. The oranges also provide a surprising source of calcium.

1 Peel and grate the carrots and place in a serving bowl.

2 Chop the orange flesh, retaining the juices and add to the carrots.

3 Put the lemon juice, olive oil, cumin and cinnamon in a jug and whisk together well. Pour over the carrots and oranges. Just before serving, mix in the chopped herbs.

4 large carrots

2 oranges, peeled and pith removed

2 teaspoons lemon juice

2 tablespoons olive oil

1 teaspoon ground cumin

1 teaspoon ground cinnamon

5 tablespoons of a mixture of finely chopped fresh sage, basil and mint

Serves 4

QUINOA SALAD

A grain of South American origin, quinoa is a useful non-wheat form of carbohydrate. Serve with leaves of romaine lettuce and garnish with shredded spring onion for a fresh green side dish.

100 g quinoa, rinsed

300 ml hot stock

50 g pine nuts

3 spring onions, chopped

1 courgette, grated

½ teaspoon turmeric

Pinch of dried oregano

Pinch of paprika

Pinch of garlic salt

1 teaspoon lemon juice

Serves 4

1 Place a medium-sized saucepan over a medium-low heat and add the quinoa. Cook, dry, for about 2 minutes, stirring occasionally, until the quinoa gives off an aroma. Then add the hot stock, turn up the heat and bring to a boil. Reduce the heat to the lowest setting, cover the pan and simmer for 20 minutes. Drain off any liquid that remains.

2 Meanwhile, heat the grill to its highest setting and toast the pine nuts for a few seconds until lightly coloured. Set aside.

3 Stir the spring onions, courgette, turmeric, dried oregano, paprika, garlic salt and lemon juice into the quinoa when it has finished cooking. Cover and leave to stand for 5 minutes.

4 Transfer the quinoa to a serving bowl to cool. Stir in the toasted pine nuts to serve, warm or cold.

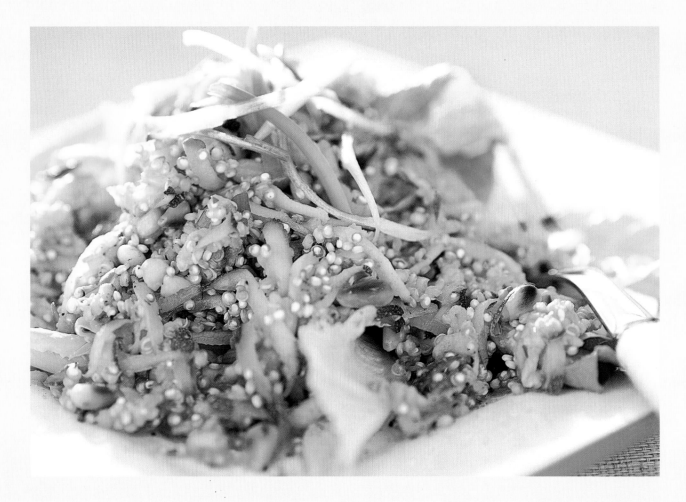

QUINOA WITH WALNUTS & ROSEMARY

Quinoa seeds have a sweet flavour and soft texture when cooked. Use them instead of pasta, bulgar wheat or couscous to create delicious gluten-free accompaniments.

1   Heat the oil in a medium-sized saucepan over medium heat and fry the onion for 2–5 minutes until it becomes translucent. Add the pepper and cook for a further 2 minutes.

2   Stir in the quinoa until well coated with the oil – it will sizzle and pop a little. Cook, stirring constantly, for 2 minutes and then add the peas, soy sauce, rosemary and 500 ml water. Bring to a boil then cover and simmer for 20 minutes.

3   Meanwhile, preheat the oven to 180°C, gas mark 4. Lay out the walnuts in a single layer on a baking tray and roast for 5 minutes.

4   When the quinoa is cooked drain off any remaining cooking liquid. Stir in the walnuts, flax oil and sesame oil and leave to stand, covered, for another 10 minutes. Serve warm.

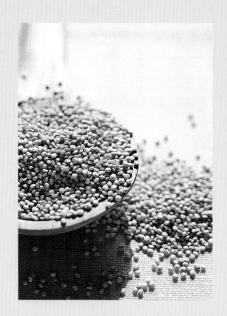

ITALIAN-STYLE QUINOA

Follow step 1 above but use 2 shallots, finely chopped, instead of the onion and omit the pepper. When you stir in the quinoa, as in step 2, add 100 g canned or bottled artichoke hearts, roughly chopped, and 1 teaspoon of the liquid from the can or jar with the water. When the quinoa is cooked, stir in 2 teaspoons chopped fresh basil, 50 g chopped sun-dried tomatoes, 2 teaspoons of the oil from the sun-dried tomatoes and 2 teaspoons flax oil. Cover and stand for 10 minutes to give the flavours a chance to develop.

---

1 tablespoon rapeseed or sunflower oil

1 small onion, finely chopped

1 red pepper, finely chopped

100 g quinoa, rinsed

100 g frozen peas

1 teaspoon soy sauce

1 teaspoon chopped fresh rosemary

50 g chopped walnuts

2 teaspoons flax oil

2 teaspoons sesame oil

Serves 4

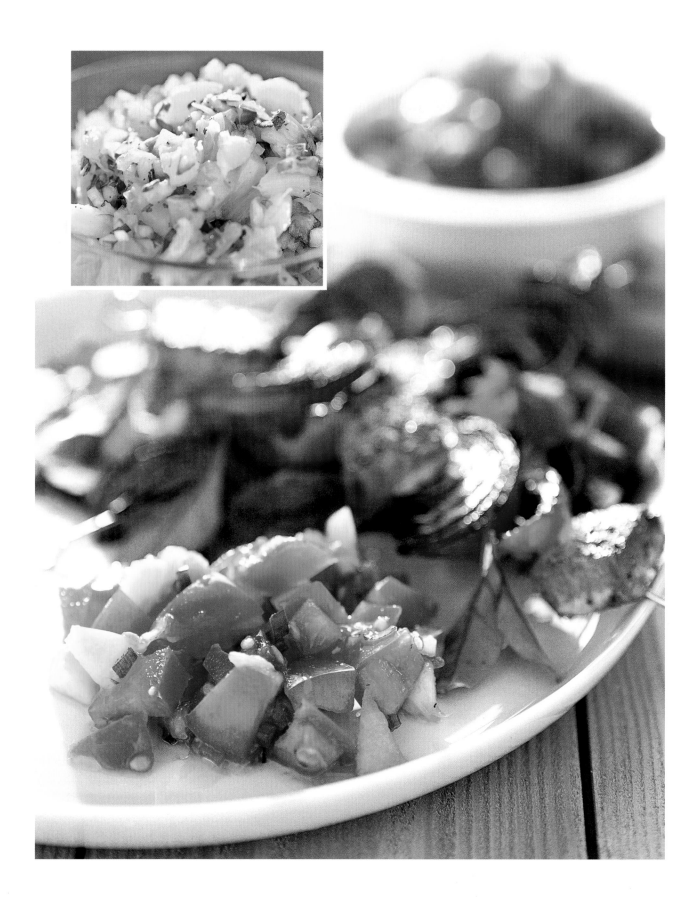

TOMATO SALSA

A tangy accompaniment that's great with well-flavoured dishes. Tomatoes are high in lycopene, another cancer-fighting nutrient.

1 Coarsely chop the tomatoes and transfer to a bowl with their juices.

2 Coarsely chop the red pepper and nectarine, peach or orange. Finely chop the spring onions. Stir all these into the tomatoes.

3 Stir in the vinegar and tomato juice and mix thoroughly. Leave to stand for at least 30 minutes at room temperature.

2 very ripe tomatoes

½ red pepper

½ nectarine, peach or orange

2 spring onions

1 teaspoon balsamic vinegar

1 teaspoon tomato juice.

Serves 4

PINEAPPLE SALSA

A low-fat, low-calorie salsa that brings the flavour of pineapple to savoury dishes – ideal served with barbecued fish, meat and vegetables.

1 Peel the pineapple, removing any 'eyes', and cut out the core; discard. Chop the flesh into small pieces and transfer to a bowl. Peel and finely chop the onion and stir it into the pineapple. Stir in the chopped herbs and lime juice.

2 Taste and then add salt and pepper, as necessary. Cover and leave to stand for at least 30 minutes at room temperature.

1 small pineapple

1 red onion

1 teaspoon finely chopped fresh sage

1 teaspoon finely chopped fresh coriander

1 teaspoon lime juice

Salt and pepper, to taste

Serves 4

HERB SALSA

A fresh-tasting, herb-packed salsa, this makes the ideal accompaniment to fish as well as plainly cooked meat and chicken.

1 Peel and finely chop the onion. Finely chop the sour dill pickle and the anchovy fillet. Mix with the oil from the tin of anchovies.

2 Stir in the cider vinegar and chopped fresh herbs. Use the salsa within 30 minutes of making.

½ onion

1 sour dill pickle

1 canned anchovy fillet

1–2 tablespoons oil from the can of anchovies

1 tablespoon cider vinegar

1 tablespoon chopped fresh chives

1 tablespoon chopped fresh parsley

1 tablespoon chopped fresh sage

Serves 2

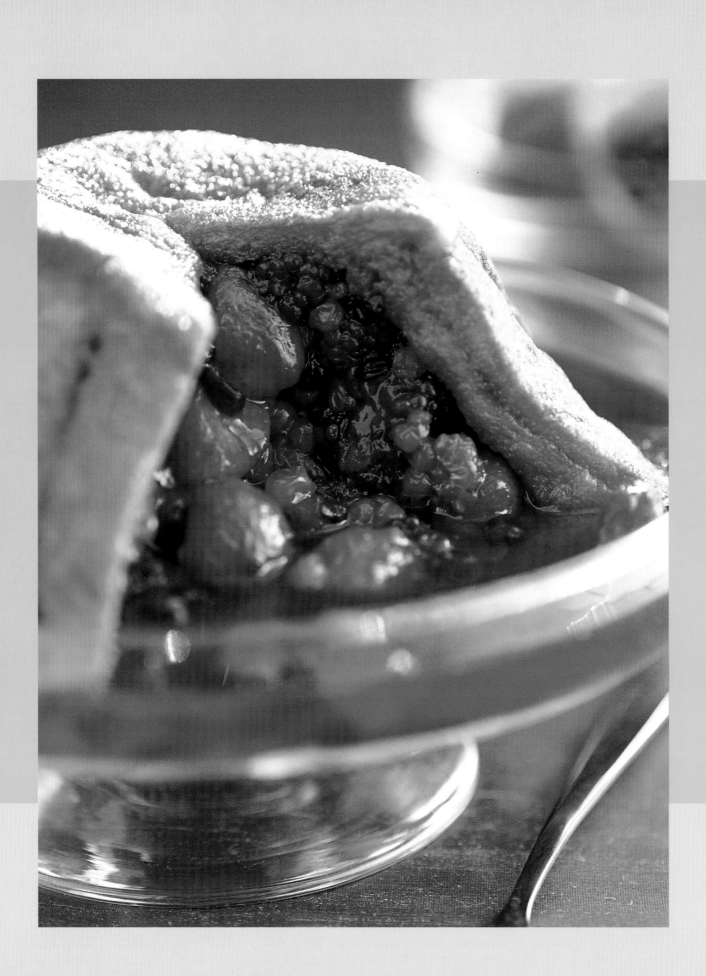

6 Sweet Treats

FRESH FRUIT DESSERTS ARE
PACKED WITH GOODNESS BUT
MANY OTHER PUDDINGS AND
BAKES CAN BE BENEFICIAL
TOO – EVEN IF IT'S IN THE
FEEL-GOOD FACTOR ALONE!

BAKED ALMOND APPLES

4 large cooking apples

Juice of ½ lemon

125 g ground almonds

110 ml apple juice or cider

4 tablespoons soft light brown sugar

½ teaspoon ground cinnamon

½ teaspoon ground mixed spice

Serves 4

A simple dessert that's a perfect combination of flavours – the almond richness, a spicy sweetness and the sharp autumnal taste of the apples. This is a great way to eat more soluble fibre.

1 Preheat oven to 180°C, gas mark 4. Core the apples. Sprinkle the lemon juice inside the apples, to prevent browning. Mix the ground almonds with 2 teaspoons of the apple juice or cider to form a thick paste. Stuff the apples with this mixture.

2 Put the apples in a baking dish in which they fit snugly. Pour the remaining apple juice or cider around the apples. Mix the brown sugar, cinnamon and ground mixed spice together in a small bowl. Sprinkle the mixture evenly over the apples.

3 Bake the apples, uncovered, for 30 minutes until the apples are soft and cooked through. Leave to cool a little before serving.

APPLE BERRY COMPOTE

3 large eating apples, peeled, cored and cut into 3 cm chunks

Juice of 1 lemon

75 g caster sugar

50 ml blackcurrant liqueur, raspberry liqueur or cranberry juice

250 g strawberries or 250 g mixed berry fruits, such as blackberries, raspberries or redcurrants

Serves 6

Berry fruits make wonderful desserts at the best of times and are high in vitamin C and flavonoids. Serve this compote with yogurt for a creamy teatime treat.

1 Place the apple chunks in a bowl and mix thoroughly with the lemon juice. Place the sugar in a medium-sized saucepan and add 100 ml water. Bring to the boil, stirring constantly, until the sugar has dissolved. Reduce the heat and simmer the syrup gently for 15 minutes.

2 Add the apple and lemon juice to the syrup and cook on a low heat. After 12 minutes, stir in the liqueur. Continue to cook for 3–4 more minutes.

3 Turn into a bowl and leave to cool. When ready to serve, mix the berries into the apples. Serve warm or cool.

CHOCOLATE BLUEBERRY TRIFLES

*Blueberries are a superior source of vitamin C and the best quality
dark chocolate is high in anti-oxidants, making this a luxury recipe
with a nutritious edge.*

1 Break the sponge fingers or ratafia biscuits into small pieces and divide
between four small individual serving dishes. Sprinkle 2 tablespoons of
sherry over each dish. Leave to stand for 20 minutes. Spoon half the
blueberries into the dishes.

2 Melt the chocolate in a bowl over a pan of simmering water then leave to
cool for about 5 minutes. Whip the cream until it forms soft peaks and fold
all but 2 tablespoons of the melted chocolate into the whipped cream.

3 Spoon the chocolate-cream into the individual dishes. Top with the
remaining blueberries and decorate with a few raspberries. Drizzle on the
reserved melted chocolate; chill. Dust with icing sugar to serve.

4 sponge fingers or 8 ratafia biscuits

120 ml sherry

150 g blueberries

150 g dark chocolate

125 ml double cream

A few raspberries, to decorate

Icing sugar, for dusting

Serves 4

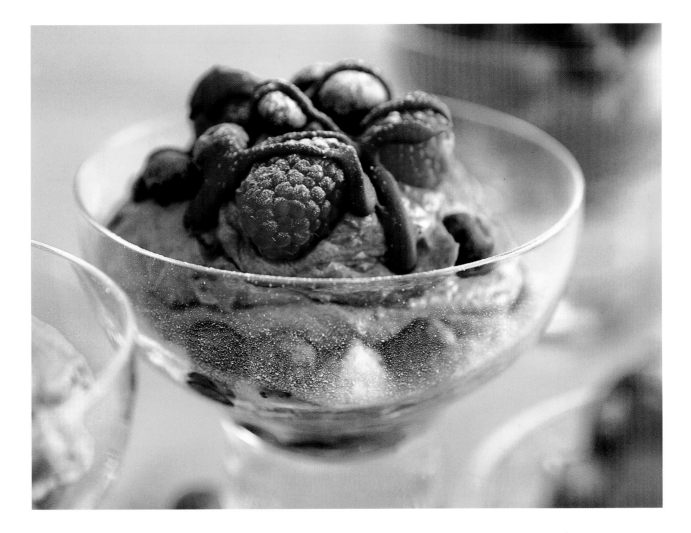

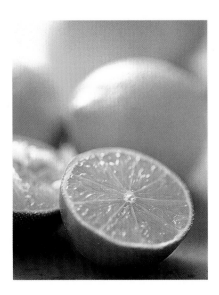

1 lemon

1 lime

1 orange

50 g caster sugar

1 teaspoon cornflour

250 g mascarpone cheese

3 tablespoons icing sugar

Butter for greasing

CITRUS CRÊPES WITH A TANGY SAUCE

This is a lovely dessert, perfectly accompanied by a tangy sauce, made with lemons, limes and orange. The crêpes are filled with high-calcium mascarpone cheese and the sauce is rich in vitamin C.

1 To make the citrus sauce, remove the zest of the lemon, lime and orange in long strips, using a vegetable peeler; transfer to a small saucepan and add 100 ml water. Squeeze the juice of half the orange into a separate bowl and set aside. Squeeze the remaining orange juice and the lemon and lime juices into a jug.

2 Place the small saucepan over a medium-high heat and bring to the boil. Boil rapidly for 3–5 minutes. Remove the pan from the heat and discard the pieces of zest. Add 25 g caster sugar, stirring well until it's dissolved. Leave to cool slightly.

3 Mix the cornflour with a teaspoon of the mixed lemon, lime and orange juices to make a smooth paste. Gradually stir the paste into the saucepan and add the rest of the mixed juices. Bring to a boil. Cook, stirring, for 2–3 minutes. Leave to cool before refrigerating for at least 1 hour.

4 To make the mascarpone filling, take the bowl containing the reserved orange juice and add the mascarpone and remaining caster sugar. Beat everything together then cover and chill for 1 hour.

5 To make the crêpes, sift the flour into large bowl. Make a well in the flour and pour in the egg. Pour in half the milk, a little at a time, beating the flour into the liquid with each addition. When all the flour is incorporated, whisk the batter until smooth. Set aside for a few minutes before adding the remaining milk and the oil. Whisk the batter until it is slightly bubbly and has the consistency of single cream. Set aside for at least 30 minutes.

6 To cook the crêpes, grease a small frying pan with the extra oil and place over a fairly high heat. Pour in enough batter to thinly coat the bottom of the pan. Cook until little bubbles break on the surface of the pancake, then turn and cook for another couple of minutes. Repeat until all the batter is used up. Separate the crêpes with sheets of greaseproof paper and set aside to cool slightly.

7   To assemble the dish, lay out each crêpe and divide the filling between them, spreading it over half of each crêpe. Fold each crepe in half over the filling and then in half again. Grease a large heatproof serving dish with the butter and arrange the crêpes in it, overlapping them if necessary. Cover and refrigerate for 1 hour

8   When ready to serve, preheat the grill to its highest setting. Dust the crêpes with the icing sugar and grill for about 2 minutes until they begin to brown at the edges and the sugar starts to bubble slightly. Heat the citrus sauce in a small pan over medium-low heat and pour over the crêpes; serve at once.

FOR THE CRÊPES

115 g plain flour

1 egg beaten

300 ml milk

1 teaspoon sunflower oil, plus extra for greasing

Serves 4

SUMMER PUDDING

This traditional English pudding is packed with summer goodness – and low in fat. Strawberries, raspberries and currants are high in vitamin C and anti-oxidant nutrients.

1   Place the berries in a large saucepan and add the sugar. Cook over a very low heat for 10 minutes until the juices run; cool. Drain the fruit, retaining the juice.

2   Trim the crusts off the bread and cut one slice to fit the bottom of a 1.4-litre pudding basin. Dip this piece into the retained juice and place in the bottom of the basin. Use more of the bread to line the sides of the basin, cutting pieces to fit as necessary and overlapping them, dipping each piece in the retained juice as you work. There should be no gaps or the juices will leak out.

3   Fill the bread-lined basin with the fruit. Cut more of the bread to fit the top, so it fits snugly inside the rim of the bowl and no fruit is exposed, dipping it in the retained juice before you put it in place. Pour any remaining juices over the bread so no white is visible and the bread is lightly moistened.

4   Place a plate that's slightly smaller than the outer edge of the bowl on top of the pudding and weigh it down with tin cans. Refrigerate overnight. To serve, turn out on to a dish.

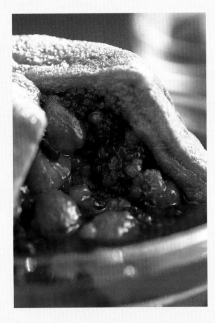

700 g of a mixture of berry fruits – strawberries, raspberries, redcurrants and blackcurrants

115 g caster sugar

10–12 slices day-old, medium-sliced white bread

Serves 6

MERINGUE NESTS WITH APRICOT FILLING

Although low in fat, the apricot purée that fills these pavlova-style meringue nests is surprisingly rich. Dried apricots are also a good source of iron, betacarotene, fibre and calcium.

3 egg whites

175 g caster sugar

1 teaspoon cornflour

1 teaspoon white wine vinegar

1 teaspoon vanilla extract

350 g dried apricots

Juice of 1 lemon

Pinch of ground cinnamon

350–400 ml cider or apple juice

4 tablespoons Greek yogurt, to serve

Sprigs of mint and orange zest curls, to decorate

Serves 4

1   Preheat the oven to 130°C, gas mark ½. Draw four 10 cm circles onto a sheet of baking parchment. Turn the baking parchment the other way up and use to cover a baking tray. Place the egg whites in a bowl and whisk until stiff. Whisk in the sugar, a spoonful at a time until the mixture forms stiff peaks. Fold in the cornflour, vinegar and vanilla extract. Spoon the mixture into the circles on the baking parchment, spreading the mixture slightly. Bake for 1¼ hours.

2   Place the apricots, lemon juice, cinnamon and 350 ml cider or apple juice in a medium-sized saucepan. Bring to a boil, cover and reduce the heat to simmer. Cook for 25–30 minutes. Remove the lid and leave to cool.

3   Transfer the contents of the pan to a food processor or liquidiser and purée. If there is not enough cooking liquid left to purée the mix adequately, add a little more cider or apple juice, a spoonful at a time.

4   Spoon the mixture into the cooked meringue nests. To serve, pour a spoonful of Greek yogurt on top of the apricot purée and decorate with orange zest curls and sprigs of mint.

CANARY ISLAND FRUIT SALAD

A delicious mixture of tropical fruits, this dessert makes a low-fat, healthy end to any meal. Packed with vitamin C, betacarotene and potassium, these fruits are also a perfect source of fibre.

Juice of 1 orange

Juice of 1 lemon

100 g runny honey

2 tablespoons orange liqueur

1 small pineapple

1 papaya

1 mango

1 banana

3 kiwi fruits

Serves 6

1   Mix together the orange juice, lemon juice, honey and orange liqueur in a small bowl.

2   Peel all the fruit. Remove and discard the core of the pineapple, the papaya seeds and mango stone. Cut the pineapple, papaya and mango into 2 cm cubes. Cut the banana into 1 cm-thick slices. Thinly slice the kiwi fruits.

3   Mix the fruit together in a large serving bowl. Stir in the juice and honey mixture. Chill for at least 2 hours before serving.

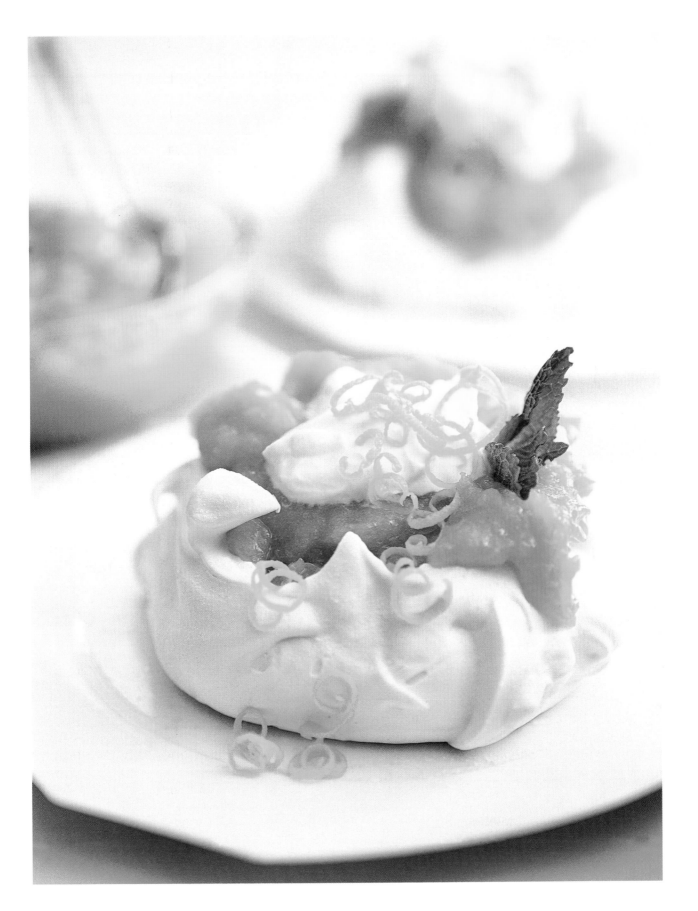

CARAMELISED FIGS

8 fresh figs

Zest and juice of 1 large orange

3 tablespoons demerara sugar

4 tablespoons Grand Marnier
or orange liqueur

250 g tub mascarpone cheese

Serves 4

A simple but elegant dessert, this is a wonderful way to eat figs. They are served with mascarpone cheese that's been flavoured with an orange liqueur. Serve plain if you're watching your waistline.

1   Cut a cross into the top of each fig, cutting down halfway into each fruit. Squeeze each one slightly at the base so that the fruit opens out and the flesh is visible inside the cut.

2   Place the figs cut-side up in a shallow baking dish and sprinkle with the orange juice and most of the zest; set aside a little for decoration. Sprinkle each fig with the sugar.

3   Preheat the grill to its highest setting. Place the dish under the grill and grill the figs for about 10 minutes until the sugar has melted and the edges of the fruit begin to caramelise.

4   Meanwhile, stir the liqueur into the mascarpone. Serve with the warm figs, drizzled with some of the cooking juices and a little of the zest.

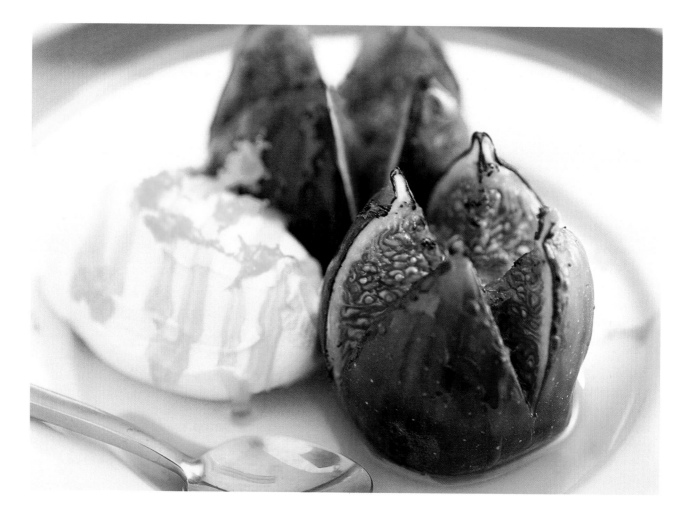

GRAPE BRULÉE PUDDING

Sweet and juicy grapes are teamed with a creamy filling to make a very rich pudding that's almost like a cheesecake. Definitely one for special occasions, this is a dish for making a day in advance.

1 Put the biscuits in a bag and crush with a rolling pin. Wash the black and green grapes separately and drain thoroughly. Pour both kinds of cream into a bowl together and whip until almost stiff.

2 Take a 2 litre flameproof serving dish and line the base with half the crushed biscuits. Add the black grapes. Top this layer with half the whipped cream.

3 Cover the cream with the rest of the crushed biscuits. Add a layer of green grapes then cover with the remaining cream. Sprinkle the sugar over the top and leave in the fridge overnight.

4 About 3½ hours before you wish to serve, heat the grill to its highest setting. Place the dish underneath and grill for 3–5 minutes, watching continuously. When the sugar has darkened and is bubbling, remove the dish and leave to cool. Refrigerate again for at least 3 hours.

225 g digestive biscuits

225 g black seedless grapes

225 g green seedless grapes

300 ml double cream

150 ml single cream

175 g demerara sugar

Serves 4

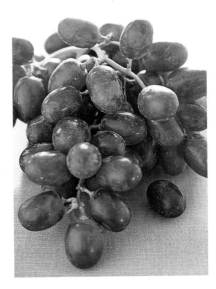

DATES IN TOFFEE BUTTERSCOTCH SAUCE

A real sweet treat, this is true comfort food, just right if you're in the mood for something indulgent. The sesame seeds are a good source of calcium.

1 Place a cast-iron skillet or heavy-based frying pan over medium-high heat. When the pan is hot, dry-fry the sesame seeds for a few seconds until they begin to colour and give off an aroma; set aside.

2 Pour the cream into a saucepan and heat over a very low heat. Put the caster and demerara sugars in another pan with 4 tablespoons water and place over medium-high heat, stirring to ensure the sugar has dissolved. Boil until the liquid turns golden and thickens a little. Remove from the heat and pour into the hot cream, a little at a time, stirring vigorously with each addition.

3 Bring the sauce to a boil for 5 minutes, stirring constantly, until it has a thick toffee-like consistency. Stir in the dates and reserved sesame seeds and cook on a low heat for 3–4 minutes. Pour into individual dishes to serve, accompanied by crème fraîche and decorated with mint leaves.

3 teaspoons sesame seeds

100 ml double cream

75 g caster sugar

1 tablespoon demerara sugar

20 fresh dates, pitted

Crème fraîche, to serve

Mint leaves, to decorate

Serves 4

CHERRY NUT FLORENTINES

These wonderful wheat-free biscuits, packed with calcium-rich nuts, will satisfy any cravings for sweet things.

Sunflower oil, for greasing

80 g sultanas

60 g flaked almonds

100 g chopped hazelnuts

100 g glacé cherries, finely chopped

160–200 ml sweetened condensed milk

100 g dark chocolate

Makes 15–20 Florentines

1 Preheat oven to 180°C, gas mark 4. Line a baking tray with greaseproof paper and brush with a little sunflower oil to prevent sticking. Mix together the sultanas, flaked almonds, chopped hazelnuts and cherries in a large bowl. Add 160 ml condensed milk and stir well. The mixture needs to have a stiff dropping consistency, so add extra milk if necessary.

2 Drop small spoonfuls of the mixture on to the prepared baking tray. Using a knife, spread them out as flat as possible, making sure there are no gaps in the mixture. Bake for 10 minutes.

3 Remove from the oven and leave to cool for 5 minutes. Using the back of a knife, draw the edges of the florentines in, to neaten their shape. Transfer, still on the sheet of greaseproof, to a cooling rack. Once cool, transfer to a fresh sheet of greaseproof paper and chill for at least 1 hour.

4 When the florentines are completely chilled, melt the chocolate in a bowl over a pan of simmering water. Turn the florentines upside down and spoon the melted chocolate over each one, smoothing it out to completely coat the back of each biscuit. Cool and chill again before serving.

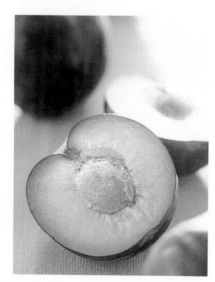

ALMOND & PLUM TART

Juicy plums and and almondy filling pack this tart. You can use any kind of plum, choose whichever is best in season. The almonds make a good contribution to essential calcium levels.

45 g butter, plus extra for greasing

375 g ready-made shortcrust pastry

100 g caster sugar

150 g ground almonds

1 teaspoon almond essence

25 g plain flour

2 eggs, beaten

4 plums, stoned and sliced

Serves 8

1 Preheat the oven to 200°C, gas mark 6. Grease a 26 cm loose-bottomed flan tin with the extra butter. Roll out the pastry thinly and use to line the tin. Lightly roll a rolling pin over the top of the pastry to remove any excess. Prick the base with a fork. Refrigerate for at least 30 minutes.

2 Place a circle of baking parchment or greaseproof paper over the base of the pastry and then place baking beans or dried beans on top of the paper. Bake blind for 15 minutes. Remove the baking beans and paper and return to the oven for another 15 minutes.

3 Reduce the oven to 180°C, gas mark 4. Put the butter, sugar, ground almonds, almond essence, flour and eggs in a large bowl and beat together until smooth. Spread over the baked pastry case.

4 Scatter the plums over the mixture and press in slightly. Bake for 40 minutes or until the pastry is golden and the filling is firm when lightly pressed. Serve warm.

BANANA DATE CRÊPES

This makes an ideal dinner-party dessert, full of healthy ingredients that will satisfy the sweetest tooth. Bananas are packed with vitamin B6 and potassium, and dates are a good source of fibre.

1   Mix together the cornflour, egg yolk, 3 tablespoons of milk and a pinch of salt in a jug. Pour the remaining milk into a medium-sized saucepan and add the sugar, butter and almond essence. Place over medium heat and bring to the boil. Remove from heat and add the cornflour mixture. Return to a low heat and stir continuously until thickened. Leave until completely cooled, then cover and chill.

2   To make the crêpes, sift the flour and salt into a mixing bowl. Make a well in the flour and pour in the egg. Pour in half the milk, a little at a time, beating the flour into the liquid with each addition. When all the flour is incorporated, whisk the batter until smooth. Set aside for a few minutes before adding the remaining milk. Whisk the batter until it is slightly bubbly with the consistency of single cream. Set aside for 30 minutes.

3   Preheat the oven to 220°C, gas mark 7. Mix the chopped dates with the ground almonds and stir into the cooled custard. Stir in the orange zest.

4   To cook the crêpes, grease a small frying pan with the oil and place over a high heat. Pour in enough batter to thinly coat the bottom of the pan. Cook until little bubbles break on the surface of the pancake then turn and cook for another couple of minutes. Repeat until all the batter is used up.

5   To assemble the dish, cut each banana in half lengthwise. Lay out the crêpes and place two banana halves plus one spoonful of the filling on each crepe. Roll up each crêpe around the bananas and place in a greased baking dish. Bake for 15 minutes until the edges of the crêpes begin to turn a golden brown.

6   Meanwhile, make the sauce. Melt the butter over a very low heat and add the sugar. When it has dissolved add the orange juice. Remove the crêpes from the oven and pour on the hot sauce. Serve hot or warm.

1 tablespoon cornflour

1 egg yolk

270 ml milk

Pinch of salt

1 tablespoon caster sugar

25 g butter

3 drops almond essence

8 fresh dates, pitted and finely chopped

4 dried dates, pitted and finely chopped

150 g ground almonds

Grated zest of 1 orange

4 bananas

FOR THE CRÊPES

60 g plain flour

Pinch of salt

1 small egg, beaten

150 ml milk

Sunflower oil, for greasing

FOR THE SAUCE

60 g butter

225 g caster sugar

100 ml orange juice

Serves 4

COCONUT CREAM PEACH PIE

Butter, for greasing

250 g ready-made shortcrust pastry

6 peaches

60 g ground rice

1 teaspoon ground cinnamon

2 tablespoons desiccated coconut

100 g caster sugar

250 ml double cream

Serves 8–10

Make the most of fresh peaches in their summertime season with this luscious pie. If you can't get decent peaches, use plums instead – you'll need 10–12, stoned and cut into slices.

1   Preheat the oven to 200°C, gas mark 6. Lightly grease a 20 cm round pie tin or shallow cake tin with the butter. Roll out the pastry and use it to line the tin. Lightly roll a rolling pin over the top of the pastry to remove any excess. Prick the base with a fork. Refrigerate for at least 30 minutes.

2   Place a circle of baking parchment or greaseproof paper over the base of the pastry and then place baking beans or dried beans on top of the paper. Bake blind in the middle of the oven for 20 minutes. Remove the baking beans and paper and bake for another 5 minutes.

3   Meanwhile, peel, stone and slice the peaches. When the pastry case is cooked, add the peach slices until the case is about two-thirds full.

4   Mix the ground rice, cinnamon, coconut, sugar and cream together in a medium-sized saucepan. Stir and leave to stand for 5 minutes. Place the pan over a low heat and bring the mixture just up to a boiling point, but do not allow to boil. Pour the mixture over the peaches. Bake the pie for 45–55 minutes or until set – a skewer, when inserted in the filling, should come out clean. Serve warm.

FIGGY CHOCOLATE NUT CAKE

100 g flaked almonds

75 g walnuts, chopped

Butter, for greasing

150 g dried figs

75 g dark chocolate

3 eggs

50 g caster sugar

150 g raisins or sultanas

150 g self-raising flour

Makes 8–10 servings

This is a delicious cake, heavy in texture and almost like a fruit bread. Made without the addition of a cooking fat, it makes a satisfying snack or even a quick, energy-packed breakfast.

1   Preheat the oven to 180°C, gas mark 4. Line a baking tray with foil and sprinkle on the nuts. Toast in the middle of the oven for 15 minutes.

2   Meanwhile, grease a 20 cm round cake tin with the butter. Chop the figs and grate or finely chop the chocolate.

3   Put the eggs and sugar in a large bowl and beat together until fluffy. Add the toasted nuts, figs, raisins and chocolate and combine well. Sift in the flour and mix gently.

4   Pour into the prepared cake tin and bake for 1 hour or until a skewer comes out clean when inserted in the middle of the cake. Leave to cool in the tin before turning out.

NO-BAKE CHOCOLATE CAKE

A sumptuous cake, rich in cancer-fighting flavonoids from the cranberries and chocolate. Use a dark chocolate with at least 70 per cent cocoa solids.

1 Put the dried cranberries in a small bowl and pour on the cranberry juice. Soak for at least 2 hours. Lightly grease a 20 cm loose-based cake tin with the extra butter.

2 Put the ginger nuts in a plastic bag and crush them with a rolling pin. Place the chocolate and butter in a bowl over a saucepan of gently simmering water and melt together, stirring occasionally.

3 Pour the cream into a separate bowl whip until it very stiff. Drain the dried cranberries and stir them into the cream. Add the walnut pieces and crushed ginger nuts. Beat in the melted chocolate.

4 Pour the whole mixture into the cake tin and smooth the top. Cover and chill for at least 6 hours. Slice to serve.

50 g dried cranberries

3 tablespoons cranberry juice

50 g butter, plus extra for greasing

225 g ginger nut biscuits

225 g dark chocolate, broken into pieces

150 ml double cream

110 g walnut pieces

Makes 8–10 servings

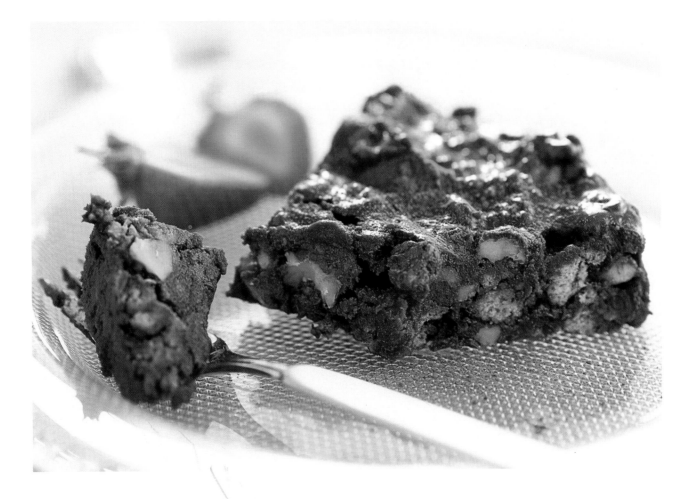

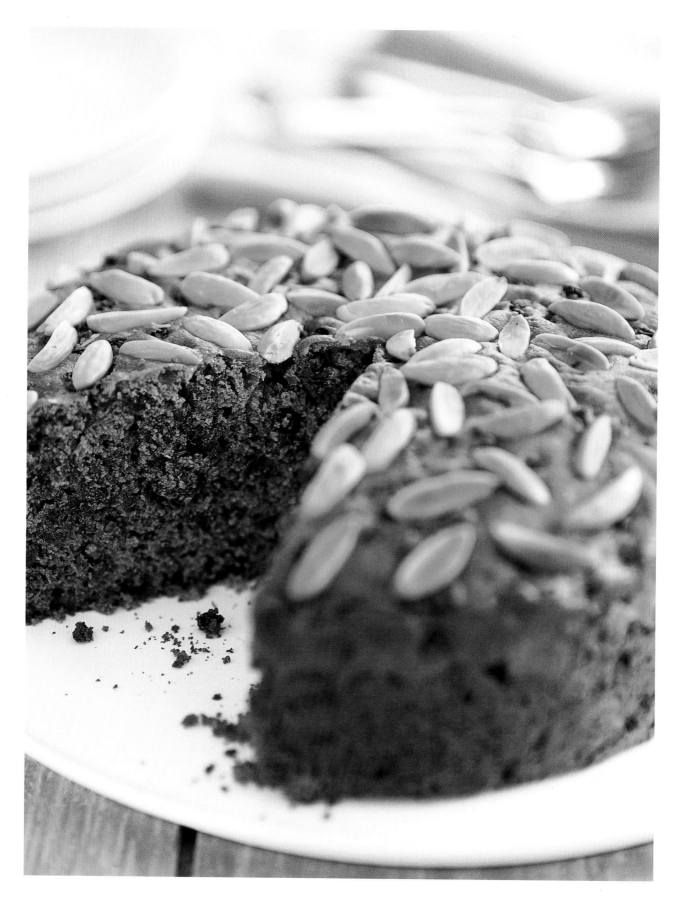

FLAPJACKS

Oats can help lower cholesterol and regulate blood sugar while the oil found in linseeds is an almost perfect balance of both the Omega 6 and Omega 3 fatty acids.

1 Preheat the oven to 190°C, gas mark 5. Grease a shallow-sided baking tin, about 25 cm square, with the extra butter. Chop the figs and apricots into small pieces and peel and grate the apple.

2 Melt the sugar, syrup and remaining butter together in a large saucepan over low heat, stirring well. Add the figs, apricots, grated apple, linseeds, oats, salt and cinnamon; stir well.

3 Pour the mixture into the prepared tin and bake in the centre of the oven for 30 minutes until golden. Leave to cool for 10 minutes then mark into squares while still in the tin. Leave to cool completely before turning out.

175 g butter, plus extra for greasing

40 g dried figs

50g dried apricots

1 eating apple

150 g demerara sugar

1 tablespoon golden syrup

2 tablespoons linseeds

350 g oats

Pinch of salt

1 teaspoon ground cinnamon

Makes about 15 squares

FRUIT CAKE

Dried fruit and nuts are sources of calcium that are often overlooked, making this cake an ideal way to help keep bones strong.

1 Heat the oven to 180°C, gas mark 4. Grease a 22 cm cake tin with the extra butter. Melt the remaining butter in a large saucepan over medium-low heat and add all the fruit, sugar, spices and juice. Add 125 ml water. Bring to boil for 1 minute and then remove from heat and leave to cool.

2 Once completely cool, transfer the boiled fruit to a large bowl and beat in the eggs. Sift in the flours and bicarbonate of soda and beat well again.

3 Pour the mixture into the prepared cake tin and sprinkle with the almonds or walnuts. Bake for 1–1½ hours until a skewer, when inserted in the cake, comes out clean.

4 Leave the cake in the oven to cool slightly then allow to cool in the tin for at least 1 hour before turning out.

125 g softened butter, plus extra for greasing

250 g sultanas

250 g currants

150 g soft light brown sugar

1 teaspoon ground cinnamon

1 teaspoon ground ginger

125 ml apple juice

2 eggs, beaten

100 g plain flour

200 g self-raising flour

1 teaspoon bicarbonate of soda

50 g slivered almonds or chopped walnuts

8–10 Servings

Women, if not on a diet, should consume around 2000 calories (KJ 8360) a day. You should eat no more than 6g salt a day and no more than 70g fat, of which the saturated fats should not exceed 20g. Don't worry if you do go over your daily limit – you can just cut back the next day. Ideally, you also need 18g fibre and 700mg calcium a day.

The nutritional information for each recipe refers to a single serving, unless otherwise stated. Optional ingredients and variation recipes are not included. The figures are intended as a guide only.

p.12 Mango & Peach Smoothie
calories 275 (KJ 1149); salt 0.3g; fat 5g; saturated fat 1g; fibre 6g; calcium 141mg

p.12 Coffee Banana Smoothie
calories 120 (KJ 502); salt 0.05g; fat 1.5g; saturated fat 0.5g; fibre 0.5g; calcium 190mg

p.13 Very Berry Smoothie
calories 307 (KJ 1283); salt 0.45g; fat 7g; saturated fat 1.5g; fibre 3g; calcium 322mg

p.14 Grilled Pink Grapefruit with Nutmeg & Maple Syrup Crust
calories 102 (KJ 426); salt 0.009g; fat 0g; saturated fat 0g; fibre 1g; calcium 34mg

p.15 Caribbean Porridge
calories 646–430 (KJ 2700–1797); salt 0.2–0.14g; fat 40–26g; saturated fat 14–9g; fibre 38–5g; calcium 73–49mg

p.17 Vanilla Granola Breakfast Trifle
calories 635 (KJ 2654); salt 0.6g; fat 28g; saturated fat 3g; fibre 6g; calcium 87mg

p.18 French-toasted Brioche with Forest Berry Sauce
calories 270 (KJ 1129); fat 8g; saturated fat 3g; fibre 2g; calcium 100mg

p.19 Carrot Breakfast Muffins
calories 250 (KJ 1045); salt 0.9g; fat 15g; saturated fat 2g; fibre 2g; calcium 100mg

p.20 Daily Loaf
calories 200–162 (KJ 836–677); salt 0.06–0.05g; fat 11–9g; saturated fat 1.5–1g; fibre 2.5–2g; calcium 104–85mg

p.21 Banana & Cottage Cheese Topped Bagels
calories 386 (KJ 1613); salt 1.5g; fat 12g; saturated fat 2g; fibre 2g; calcium 162mg

p.21 Smoked Salmon & Quark with Onion Bagels
calories 290 (KJ 1212); salt 2.8g; fat 3g; saturated fat 0.5g; fibre 1g; calcium 170mg

p.22 Oven-baked Hash Brown with Tomato Gratin
calories 260 (KJ 1087); salt 0.7g; fat 10g; saturated fat 3g; fibre 4g; calcium 212mg

p.23 Springtime Herb Frittata
calories 354–177 (KJ 11480–740); salt 0.7–0.35g; fat 28–14g; saturated fat 11–6g; fibre 0–0g; calcium 136–68mg

p.25 Baked Eggs & Mushrooms in Ham Crisps
calories 345 (KJ 1442); salt 1.2g; fat 18g; saturated fat 5g; fibre 4g; calcium 163mg

p.25 Creamy Scrambled Eggs with Smoked Trout
calories 350 (KJ 1463); salt 1.2g; fat 29g; saturated fat 13g; fibre 0g; calcium 106mg

p.28 Carrot & Orange Soup
calories 129 (KJ 539); salt 1g; fat 6g; saturated fat 1g; fibre 3g; calcium 47mg

p.29 Yellow Cauliflower Soup with Crusty Croutons
calories 348 (KJ 1455); salt 0.8g; fat 22g; saturated fat 6g; fibre 3g; calcium 353mg

p.30 Mushroom Soup with Miso
calories 81–61 (KJ 338–255); salt 0.9–0.7g; fat 5–4g; saturated fat 0.7–0.5g; fibre 2–1g; calcium 20–15mg

p.31 Easy Lentil Soup
calories 245 (KJ 1024); salt 0.7g; fat 5g; saturated fat 0.7g; fibre 4g; calcium 49mg

p.31 Pea & Broccoli Soup
calories 210–156 (KJ 878–652); salt 1–0.7g; fat 11–9g; saturated fat 2–1g; fibre 7–5g; calcium 66–49mg

p.32 Barley Bean Soup
calories 200 (KJ 836); salt 0.8g; fat 7.5g; saturated fat 2.5g; fibre 3g; calcium 114mg

p.33 Scarlet Soup
calories 212–160 (KJ 886–669); salt 0.8–0.56g; fat 4.5–3g; saturated fat 0.7–0.5g; fibre 4–3g; calcium 51–38mg;

p.33 Smoked Tofu Chowder
calories 235–160 (KJ 982–669); salt 1.7g; fat 10–7g; saturated fat 3–2g; fibre 4–3g; calcium 285–230mg

p.34 Mediterranean Fish Soup
calories 250 (KJ 1045); salt 3g; fat 8g; saturated fat 1g; fibre 2g; calcium 131mg

p.34 Fennel & Radicchio Salad
calories 277 (KJ 1158); salt 0.9g; fat 29g; saturated fat 3g; fibre 2g; calcium 43mg

p.36 Charred Nectarines
calories 210; (KJ 878); salt 0.05g; fat 18g; saturated fat 2g; fibre 2g; calcium 15mg

p.37 Watercress & Avocado Salad with Pitta Bread & Humus
calories 640 (KJ 2675); salt 1.4g; fat 38g; saturated fat 6g; fibre 9g; calcium 220mg

p.37 Bean Burritos
calories 500 (KJ 2090); salt 2.5g; fat 7g; saturated fat 2g; fibre 13g; calcium 250mg

p.38 Warm Salad with Tofu Parmesan
calories 270 (KJ 1129); salt 0.4g; fat 22g; saturated fat 5g; fibre 2g; calcium 400mg

p.39 Tofu Mayonnaise Open Sandwich
calories 250 (KJ 1045); salt 1.1g; fat 16g; saturated fat 2g; fibre 1g; calcium 600mg

p.40 Mozzarella Ciabatta Bites
calories 500 (KJ 2090); salt 1.2g; fat 23g; saturated fat 11g; fibre 2g; calcium 557mg

p.41 Gorgonzola, Watercress and Fig Salad
calories 320 (KJ 1338); salt 0.9g; fat 28g; saturated fat 10g; fibre 2g; calcium 236mg

p.41 Goat's Cheese with Baby Spinach and Olives
calories 180 (KJ 752); salt 1g; fat 11g; saturated fat 5g; fibre 1g; calcium 151mg

p.42 Salmon Cake Hors d'Oeuvres
calories 145 (KJ 606); salt 4.4g; fat 8g; saturated fat 1g; fibre 0g; calcium 18mg

p.43 Smoked Mackerel Appetiser
calories 210 (KJ 878); salt 1g; fat 18g; saturated fat 4g; fibre 0g; calcium 24mg

p.43 Chicken Liver Antipasti
calories 250–170 (KJ 1045–710); salt 1.1–0.8g; fat 13–9g; saturated fat 4–3g; fibre 1–0.7g; calcium 63–42mg

p.46 Feta Cheese Parcels
calories 490 (KJ 2048); salt 4.7g; fat 30g; saturated fat 18g; fibre 0g; calcium 400mg

p.47 Broccoli, Broad Bean & Feta Salad
calories 270 (KJ 1129); salt 2g; fat 22g; saturated fat 9g; fibre 4g; calcium 215mg

p.48 Chickpeas & Spinach with Garlic Rice
calories 450 (KJ 1881); salt 1g; fat 10g; saturated fat 1g; fibre 10g; calcium 190mg

p.48 Pesto Parmesan Mushrooms
calories 460 (KJ 1923); salt 0.8g; fat 41g; saturated fat 8g; fibre 1.5g; calcium 260mg

p.49 Yellow Peppers with Turmeric Cauliflower & Parmesan
calories 174 (KJ 727); salt 0.4g; fat 10g; saturated fat 5g; fibre 4g; calcium 182mg

p.50 Prawn Pasta
calories 535 (KJ 2236); salt 2.3g;
fat 6g; saturated fat 1g; fibre 4g;
calcium 126mg

p.50 Salmon Cakes
calories 360 (KJ 1505); salt 1.3g;
fat 17g; saturated fat 3g; fibre 1g;
calcium 123mg

p.51 Mediterranean Fish
calories 365 (KJ 1526); salt 1.2g;
fat 22g; saturated fat 4g; fibre 2g;
calcium 75mg

**p.52 Grilled Herrings with
Orange Salsa**
calories 465 (KJ 1944); salt 0.15g;
fat 37g; saturated fat 7g; fibre 2g;
calcium 75mg

p.52 Eastern Sole
calories 165 (KJ 690); salt 0.7g;
fat 4g; saturated fat 0.5g; fibre 0g;
calcium 54mg

p.53 Slightly Spicy Fish Goujons
calories 350 (KJ 1463); salt 0.5g;
fat 10g; saturated fat 1.5g;
fibre 1g; calcium 75mg

**p.54 Warm Mackerel Salad with
Potatoes & Olives**
calories 735 (KJ 3072); salt 3.5g;
fat 58g; saturated fat 11g;
fibre 1.5g; calcium 80mg

p.55 Cod in Dill Sauce
calories 260 (KJ 1087); salt 0.5g;
fat 13g; saturated fat 2g; fibre
0.5g; calcium 91mg

p.55 Flash-Fried Peppered Tuna
calories 200 (KJ 836); salt 2.5g;
fat 6g; saturated fat 2g; fibre 1g;
calcium 112mg

p.56 Charred Sesame Chicken
calories 285 (KJ 1191); salt 0.3g;
fat 21g; saturated fat 4g; fibre 1g;
calcium 111mg

p.56 Orangey Chicken
calories 235 (KJ 982); salt 0.3g;
fat 6.5g; saturated fat 2g; fibre 0g;
calcium 18mg

p.58 Turkey Stir Fry
calories 325 (KJ 1358); salt 1.3g;
fat 17g; saturated fat 3g; fibre 4g;
calcium 104mg

**p.59 Marinated Skewered
Turkey**
calories 450 (KJ 1881); salt 0.7g;
fat 5g; saturated fat 1.5g; fibre 2g;
calcium 90mg

**p.59 Pork Escalopes with Honey
& Pecans**
calories 525 (KJ 2195); salt 0.6g;
fat 34g; saturated fat 6g;
fibre 1.5g; calcium 44mg

p.60 Lamb & Halloumi Kebabs
calories 676 (KJ 2826); salt 4g; fat
44g; saturated fat 24g; fibre 2g;
calcium 450mg

**p.61 Lemon Grass Beef with
Pak Choi**
calories 345 (KJ 1442); salt 3.5g;
fat 21g; saturated fat 5g;
fibre 1.5g; calcium 107mg

**p.64 Ricotta & Mushroom
Cannelloni**
calories 740 (KJ 3093); salt 2.3g;
fat 40g; saturated fat 20g; fibre
4g; calcium 760mg

p.65 Lentils & Red Pepper Pasta
calories 720 (KJ 3010); salt 0.4g;
fat 13g; saturated fat 4g; fibre
10g; calcium 216mg

**p.67 Risotto-stuffed Red
Peppers with Walnuts & Olives**
calories 500 (KJ 2090) salt 2.2g;
fat 26g; saturated fat 8g; fibre 5g;
calcium 235mg

**p.68 Risotto with Mushrooms,
Broad Beans & Sage**
calories 378 (KJ 1580); salt 1.2g;
fat 11g; saturated fat 7g; fibre 2g;
calcium 33mg

p.69 Nutty Brown Rice Pilau
calories 630–420 (KJ 2633–1756);
salt 0.6–0.5g; fat 23–15g;
saturated fat 3–2g; fibre 7–5g;
calcium 80–53mg

p.69 Egyptian Lentil Pilau
calories 420 (KJ 1756); salt 0.5g;
fat 8g; saturated fat 1g; fibre 7g;
calcium 175mg

p.70 Mushroom Stroganoff
calories 560 (KJ 2341); salt 0.6g;
fat 10g; saturated fat 2.5g;
fibre 6g; calcium 102mg

**p.70 Coconut Tofu with Peanut
Spinach**
calories 535 (KJ 2247); salt 0.4g;
fat 49g; saturated fat 3g; fibre 1g;
calcium 696mg

p.72 Grilled Fish Florentine
calories 370 (KJ 1547); salt 1.6g;
fat 22g; saturated fat 13g; fibre 3g;
calcium 552mg

p.72 Crusty Halibut
calories 440 (KJ 1839); salt 1.3g;
fat 35g; saturated fat 9g; fibre 1g;
calcium 57mg

p.73 Smoked Haddock Fish Pie
calories 790 (KJ 3302); salt 6g;
fat 24g; saturated fat 14g; fibre 6g;
calcium 270mg

**p.74 Griddled Salmon with
Parsley Sauce**
calories 325 (KJ 1358); salt 0.35g;
fat 26g; saturated fat 4g; fibre 45g;
calcium 36mg

p.74 Crunchy Filo Salmon
calories 300 (KJ 1254); salt 0.4g;
fat 17g; saturated fat 3g; fibre 0g;
calcium 34mg

**p.76 Roast Trout with Almonds
& Herbs**
calories 400 (KJ 1672); salt 0.4g;
fat 26g; saturated fat 3g; fibre 2g;
calcium 116mg

p.77 Prawn Paella
calories 390 (KJ 1630); salt 3.5g;
fat 11g; saturated fat 2g; fibre 3g;
calcium 153mg

**p.78 Scallops with White Wine
& Parsley**
calories 560 (KJ 2341); salt 0.4g;
fat 8g; saturated fat 1g; fibre 3g;
calcium 57mg

**p.80 Moroccan Chicken with
Couscous**
calories 700 (KJ 2926); salt 0.9g;
fat 31g; saturated fat 7g; fibre 2g;
calcium 76mg

p.81 Chicken with Lentil Sauce
calories 350 (KJ 1463); salt 0.5g;
fat 10g; saturated fat 4g; fibre 5g;
calcium 103mg

p.81 Baked Citrus Chicken
calories 360 (KJ 1505); salt 0.5g;
fat 14g; saturated fat 4g; fibre 1g;
calcium 54mg

**p.82 Cider Chicken with
Tarragon**
calories 425 (KJ 1776); salt 0.5g;
fat 16g; saturated fat 4g;
fibre 1.5g; calcium 58mg

p.83 Turkey Puff Pie
calories 650 (KJ 2712); salt 1.6g;
fat 35g; saturated fat 3g; fibre 4g;
calcium 122mg

**p.84 Roast Duck with Peaches
& Ginger**
calories 450 (KJ 1881); salt 3.2g;
fat 15g; saturated fat 5g; fibre 3g;
calcium 48mg

**p.85 Duck Pancakes with
Chutney**
calories 680 (KJ 2842); salt 3.6g;
fat 30g; saturated fat 9g; fibre 3g;
calcium 210mg

**p.86 Venison with Root
Vegetables**
calories 660 (KJ 2759); salt 0.4g;
fat 20g; saturated fat 4g; fibre 4g;
calcium 48mg

p.87 Pot-roast Pork Tenderloin
calories 290 (KJ 1212); salt 2.3g;
fat 11g; saturated fat 4g; fibre 3g;
calcium 68mg

**p.87 Pork Chops with
Artichokes & Olives**
calories 350 (KJ 1463); salt 0.4g;
fat 17g; saturated fat 5g; fibre 2g;
calcium 140mg

p.88 Rösti Pork
calories 460 (KJ 1923); salt 0.4g;
fat 18g; saturated fat 6g; fibre 4g;
calcium 160mg

p.89 Lamb Tagine with Apricots
calories 620 (KJ 2592); salt 0.9g;
fat 24g; saturated fat 9g; fibre 6g;
calcium 102mg

p.90 Lamb Koftas
calories 350 (KJ 1463); salt 0.4g;
fat 21g; saturated fat 8g; fibre 1g;
calcium 25mg

p.90 Lamb Cassoulet
calories 690 (KJ 2884); salt 2.4g; fat 25g; saturated fat 10g; fibre 16g; calcium 213mg

p.92 Beery Beef with Root Vegetables
calories 430 (KJ 1797); salt 1.4g; fat 14g; saturated fat 7g; fibre 3g; calcium 83mg

p.93 Skillet Steak with Asia Pacific Noodles
calories 300 (KJ 1254); salt 1.2g; fat 6g; saturated fat 1.5g; fibre 2g; calcium 40mg

p.96 Braised Celery with Almonds
calories 133 (KJ 556); salt 0.5g; fat 13g; saturated fat 1g; fibre 1g; calcium 52mg

p.96 Braised Fennel & Onion
calories 60 (KJ 251); salt 1g; fat 3g; saturated fat 0.5g; fibre 2g; calcium 25mg

p.97 Armenian Potatoes
calories 350 (KJ 1463); salt 0.07g; fat 23g; saturated fat 3g; fibre 3g; calcium 13mg

p.98 Green & White Salad
calories 283–242 (KJ 1183–1012); salt 1.1–0.8g; fat 28–19g; saturated fat 3–2g; fibre 11–7.5g; calcium 137–91mg

p.99 Butter Beans in Creamy Mustard Sauce
calories 590 (KJ 2466); salt 1.7g; fat 44g; saturated fat 22g; fibre 7g; calcium 244mg

p.99 Lemon Sage Peas
calories 175 (KJ 732); salt 0.3g; fat 12g; saturated fat 7g; fibre 5g; calcium 23mg

p.100 Chickpea Mash
calories 184 (KJ 769); salt 0.4g; fat 12g; saturated fat 2g; fibre 4g; calcium 40mg

p.100 Cauliflower with Pecans
calories 220 (KJ 920); salt 0.6g; fat 17g; saturated fat 2g; fibre 4g; calcium 134mg

p.101 Broccoli in Black Bean Sauce
calories 125 (KJ 523); salt 0.5g; fat 10g; saturated fat 1g; fibre 2g; calcium 60mg

p.101 Colourful Cabbage Salad
calories 107–80 (KJ 447–334); salt 0.3–0.2g; fat 7–5g; saturated fat 1–1g; fibre 3–2g; calcium 55–40mg

p.102 Shredded Sesame Cabbage
calories 110 (KJ 460); salt 0.5g; fat 7g; saturated fat 1g; fibre 3g; calcium 51mg

p.102 Roast Carrot & Beetroot
calories 120 (KJ 502); salt 0.3g; fat 9g; saturated fat 1g; fibre 3g; calcium 30mg

p.103 Citrus Carrot Salad
calories 100 (KJ 418); salt 0.3g; fat 6g; saturated fat 1g; fibre 3g; calcium 50mg

p.104 Quinoa Salad
calories 190 (KJ 794); salt 0.6g; fat 10g; saturated fat 1g; fibre 2g; calcium 60mg

p.105 Quinoa with Walnuts & Rosemary
calories 250 (KJ 1045); salt 0.6g; fat 16g; saturated fat 2g; fibre 2g; calcium 44mg

p.107 Tomato Salsa
calories 30 (KJ 125); salt 0.2g; fat 0.5g; saturated fat 0g; fibre 1.5g; calcium 16mg

p.107 Pineapple Salsa
calories 40 (KJ 167); salt 0.2g; fat 0g; saturated fat 0g; fibre 1g; calcium 20mg

p.107 Herb Salsa
calories 70 (KJ 293); salt 0.2g; fat 6g; saturated fat 1g; fibre 0g; calcium 12mg

p.110 Baked Almond Apples
calories 330 (KJ 1379); salt 0.02g; fat 17g; saturated fat 1g; fibre 5g; calcium 84mg

p.110 Apple Berry Compote
calories 100 (KJ 418); salt 0.02g; fat 0g; saturated fat 0g; fibre 1.5g; calcium 9mg

p.111 Chocolate Blueberry Trifles
calories 410 (KJ 1714); salt 0.1g; fat 26g; saturated fat 16g; fibre 1g; calcium 50mg

p.112 Citrus Crêpes with a Tangy Sauce
calories 530 (KJ 2215); salt 0.6g; fat 35g; saturated fat 21g; fibre 1g; calcium 200mg

p.113 Summer Pudding
calories 223 (KJ 932); salt 0.6g; fat 1g; saturated fat 0g; fibre 2g; calcium 74mg

p.114 Meringue Nests with Apricot Filling
calories 373 (KJ 1559); salt 0.2g; fat 2g; saturated fat 1g; fibre 5g; calcium 95mg

p.114 Canary Island Fruit Salad
calories 155 (KJ 648); salt 0.01g; fat 0.5g; saturated fat 0g; fibre 3g; calcium 41mg

p.116 Caramelised Figs
calories 410 (KJ 1714); salt 0.07g; fat 30g; saturated fat 19g; fibre 1.5g; calcium 103mg

p.117 Grape Brulée Pudding
calories 916 (KJ 3829); salt 0.9g; fat 55g; saturated fat 32g; fibre 2g; calcium 140mg

p.117 Dates in Toffee Butterscotch Sauce
calories 250 (KJ 1045); salt 0.03g; fat 14g; saturated fat 8g; fibre 1g; calcium 44mg

p.118 Cherry Nut Florentines
calories 170–127 (KJ 711–531); salt 0.5–0.4g; fat 9.5–7g; saturated fat 2–2g; fibre 1–0.7g; calcium 60–45mg

p.118 Almond & Plum Tart
calories 450 (KJ 1881); salt 0.7g; fat 30g; saturated fat 9g; fibre 2g; calcium 100mg

p.119 Banana Date Crêpes
calories 828 (KJ 3461); salt 1g; fat 45g; saturated fat 16g; fibre 4g; calcium 206mg

p.120 Coconut Cream Peach Pie
calories 400–320 (KJ 1672–1338); salt 0.4–0.3g; fat 26–20g; saturated fat 14–11g; fibre 2–1.5g; calcium 52–41mg

p.120 Figgy Chocolate Nut Cake
calories 406–325 (KJ 1697–1358); salt 0.3–0.2g; fat 19–15g; saturated fat 3–2.5g; fibre 3.6–2.8g; calcium 137–110mg

p.121 No-bake Chocolate Cake
calories 520–416 (KJ 2174–1739); salt 0.4–0.3g; fat 36–29g; saturated fat 16–13g; fibre 1–0.8g; calcium 74–59mg

p.123 Flapjacks
calories 250 (KJ 1045); salt 0.5g; fat 13g; saturated fat 6g; fibre 2g; calcium 37mg

p.123 Fruit Cake
calories 555–444 (KJ 2320–1856); salt 0.5–0.4g; fat 19–15g; saturated fat 9–7g; fibre 3–2g; calcium 120–96mg

Index

ACKNOWLEDGEMENTS

Nutritional analysis: Fiona Hunter
Production: Nigel Reed
IT: Paul Stradling